HEALTHY AGING OVER 60

7 SIMPLE STEPS TO INCREASE VITALITY, BE MORE ENERGETIC, AND FEEL YOUNGER

DAVID D MCCRAY

CONTENTS

INTRODUCTION

> *"Don't worry about getting old, worry about thinking old.*
>
> — SUBHASH SHARMA

The average life expectancy is just over 72-years-old, globally, in 2022. That's an additional 42-years compared to an original life expectancy of less than 30-years (Roser et al., 2019). The increase in an average person's life expectancy can be attributed to many factors. In the past two centuries, rapid progress and advancements in science have helped humanity realize that they can achieve more than they originally believed in their lifetimes. Achievements don't have to be big or life-changing, like becoming an astronaut or president. Taking time to nurture your mind and body's well-being and cultivating your relationships with the people in your life that you care about is just as important, even if it isn't often recognized as such.

A person's average life expectancy in the United States in 2019 was 78.9-years-old. This is an additional 18.9 years higher than the average life expectancy of Americans in the 1950s, when you could expect to live for about 60 years (Roser et al., 2019). It almost makes sense why they thought your life was over at the tender age of 30 in 1950. You would have already lived half your life. That's both shocking and motivating because it means that, in the modern world, your life isn't over the minute you hit your 40s. Essentially, you can live twice as long as your ancestors; however, you need to put in the work to take care of your mental and physical health as you get older.

WHY THIS BOOK?

There may be various reasons why you've decided to learn more about anti-aging and resetting your biological clock. The fear of dying is a common reason for many people to start looking for ways to improve their health as they get older. Perhaps you're looking to decrease the chances of your health deteriorating or want to avoid illnesses that often occur as you age. These illnesses typically include high blood pressure, respiratory diseases, or even arthritis, to name a few. You may even be looking for a way to improve your overall health and well-being because you want to live longer for reasons such as being able to spend more time with the people you care about; or maybe you just want to enjoy your life now that you have the knowledge and experience that you didn't have during the first 20-years of your life.

Many people start to worry about their health as they get older. Frankly, it's a normal response to realizing you're not as young as you used to be. However, this realization often occurs at different times in a person's life and can be triggered by many things. After you've reached this realization, you may even start getting angry that you didn't try to improve your health earlier, or you may feel upset because you listened to the people in your life that discouraged you instead of doing your thing. Your anger is valid, but I need you to remember that it's never too late to become the healthiest version of yourself.

The tips and strategies in this guide have been specifically included because they can be implemented regardless of your age. What matters while you work through this book is that you are looking to improve your life and are willing to put in the effort needed to implement the knowledge and strategies contained here? Whether you are retired, close to retirement, live alone or with your children, this book is perfect if you enjoy feeling like you've accomplished something that will improve your life and well-being. This guide is also great for those who enjoy spending time with friends, family, and their local community. You don't need to be a social butterfly, but social relationships are important even if you want to remain independent as you get older. I aim to provide you with everything you need to know to achieve your goals.

The Benefits of Reading This Book

Upon completion of this guide, you will have gained an in-depth understanding of the aging process. Additionally, you will have learned about different—yet effective—strategies that can help you slow down physical deterioration and cognitive decline that normally occurs as you get older. Remember that your current age doesn't matter. You will be able to not only apply everything that you learn here almost immediately after reading this guide, but you'll also be able to integrate these tips and strategies in a way that suits your unique lifestyle and allows you to join the ranks of other SuperAgers.

SUPERAGERS

The information I discuss throughout this book is based on the habits of SuperAgers. Have you ever met someone who acts or looks as though they're in their 30s, maybe 40s, but then tell you they're actually 60 or 70-something years old? These people are known as SuperAgers, and no, most of them aren't getting surgery or using magic to keep themselves looking and feeling young. A SuperAger is someone who is in their 70s or 80s (although they can be younger), who feels younger than their actual age and has the mental and physical health of an individual who is much younger than them.

Individuals that are considered to be SuperAgers embrace challenges and leave their comfort zones to achieve their goals. Fortunately, you don't have to practice the habits of SuperAgers from an early age to reap the same benefits. You can start at any time, but you have to be committed to achieve what you set out to do, even though it'll take time before you start seeing results. As you work through this guide, I want you to remember that the healthiest version of yourself will look different when compared to others, but that doesn't mean you aren't healthy or living your best life.

The Habits of SuperAgers

The content of this guide covers various topics that fall under improving your mental or physical health. In chapter one, you will build a foundation for anti-aging by gaining an understanding of the science behind aging. The chapters that follow will contain more practical content. I have used a combination of methods and strategies throughout this guide that fall under the four main habits of SuperAgers. These habits include

- **an active lifestyle:** The importance of exercise is often emphasized by healthcare professionals and the media, but there's a reason for that. When you exercise, you take in more air, increasing your oxygen levels so that your body can perform optimally. You also improve your muscle strength—decreasing your risk of falling as you get older—and lowering your risk of developing serious age-related illnesses. Chapters three and five will explain how you can use supplements and exercise to improve your physical and mental health, while also managing your stress.

- **challenging yourself:** While it's important to remain physically active as you get older, you also need to challenge your mind. The brain is a muscle, and it needs to be stimulated and exercised. Chapters two, four, and six will explain the uses and importance of positive psychology, brain health, and grounding in more detail. Essentially, pushing yourself outside your comfort zone and learning new skills challenges your brain, allowing it to engage in a way that it hasn't done before.
- **nurturing your relationships:** Your relationships with the people in your life are important. The media often paints getting older as a lonely journey, but you aren't alone! You don't have to isolate yourself or stop living your life because you feel like only young people should go to certain events or do certain things. Chapter seven will explain the importance of your social connections and how you can build meaningful relationships despite your age.
- **indulging in moderation:** Improving your health and well-being doesn't mean you have to stop eating chocolate, avoid carbohydrates and

alcohol, or be busy every day. Engaging in an activity that makes you happy is crucial for your well-being; what matters is that you don't over do it. I think we can all agree that eating only sweets for every meal isn't the healthiest decision, but that's why moderation is so important. I will discuss indulgence throughout the book, as it does apply to multiple sections.

Who Are These SuperAgers?

You probably already look up to people who appear to have aged gracefully with little to no effort in both your daily life and community, as well as in more well-known places like Hollywood. Now you know that these individuals are also called SuperAgers, but you may be wondering who exactly these people are?

Before moving on to some more well-known Super-Agers, I want to discuss the woman who holds the title of the world's oldest human being. Kane Tanaka, born in Japan, died at 119-years-old. She may not have specifically stated she was a SuperAger or followed a specific set of rules, but her lifestyle essentially fulfilled the key habits of a typical SuperAger. While she did indulge in eating chocolate and drinking soda, Kane Tanaka also had a healthy diet that consisted of fish and vegetables. She kept her body moving and worked until she was 103-years-old. Mentally, she ensured that her brain was constantly being engaged by working on math problems and playing board games. Kane Tanaka is a great example of an average citizen who is also a SuperAger (Roberts, 2022).

Additionally, Hollywood actors are a great example because their job requirements essentially fall in line with the habits of SuperAgers like Kane Tanaka. Yes, famous actors have the money to get plastic surgery or botox as they get older, but many also engage in Super-Ager habits, and not because it's a fad. Their jobs require them to take care of themselves—physically and mentally—if they want to get good roles. This includes eating healthy and exercising, but that doesn't stop them from indulging either. Actors also have to keep their minds sharp because they need to memorize new lines, imitate certain behaviors, and even learn skills specific to a role, like horse riding, fencing, or dancing.

Actors and actresses put in the effort to purposefully take care of their well-being while also enjoying their lives, but who exactly are some of these Hollywood SuperAgers? Salma Hayek (56-years-old), Halle Berry (56-years-old), Keanu Reeves (58-years-old), Andy Samberg (44-years-old), Patrick Stewart (81-years-old), Paul Rudd (53-years-old), and Michelle Yeoh (60-years-old) are great examples of SuperAgers because many of them are mentally—or look physically—younger than their age. This is beneficial for these actors, as it opens up numerous roles that they can play despite getting older. It's also inspiring because it shows you that your age doesn't mean you have to stop living your life or doing things that make you happy.

Before we had the information and knowledge we do today—which I will discuss in this guide—it was difficult for many people to work on improving their mental and physical health as they got older. Especially due to how you were expected to act once you reached a certain age. At 70-years-old, I still feel like I'm only in my 30s, but I understand the fears and struggles that accompany getting older. That's why I wrote this book. I am here to guide you on your journey to anti-aging.

CALL TO ACTION

While you won't see results overnight, it is possible for you to continue enjoying your life as you get older, feel more energetic, and improve your vitality. So go ahead and turn the page so that you can get started on your journey to discovering the secrets of resetting your biological clock and reversing the effects of aging.

1

THE SCIENCE BEHIND AGING

Your body is made up of cells, but these cells don't last forever. Just like a machine whose parts need to be oiled and cared for as they get older, the cells in our bodies experience wear and tear that cause their structure to decline, affecting their ability to function properly. However, you can't replace damaged parts in your body like you can in a machine. As such, you need to provide your mind and body with the right care to ensure that it has what it needs to function at its best.

Before you start to panic, let me reassure you that you don't need a science degree to understand this chapter. I have provided you with all the information that you need to create a foundation for the anti-aging tips and strategies that are discussed throughout this guide.

Having a basic understanding of *how* aging works will also help you adapt these strategies in a way that suits your lifestyle and anti-aging goals.

One thing that I think many of us are aware of is that everyone ages differently. Aubrey, an 82-year-old woman, enjoys telling people who ask about her age, that she is actually 10-years-old because she still feels as though she is a young woman. She acts like one, too. Gardening, community projects, and spending time with her family are only a few of the ways that she stays active. Even her husband Nick, an 85-year-old man, is active. He likes to joke that he feels like he is busier now than before he retired. The couple tries their best to look after their health by eating right, maintaining a healthy weight, and staying as physically and mentally active as possible. Although this doesn’t mean that they don't also enjoy themselves every now and then either. Additionally, their genetics may be playing a role in how they are aging. Nick’s parents lived until the ages of 90 and 95, while Aubrey's mother passed away at 101.

Many factors play a role in how a person ages and their life expectancy. As such, two types of aging are used to explain a number of aging theories. I will discuss the most popular theories in this chapter, as they are commonly combined to explain the aging process.

Before we move on to learning about the theories of how aging works, let's first discuss whether you *can* actually increase your life expectancy.

INCREASING YOUR LIFE EXPECTANCY

The average global life expectancy has increased dramatically in recent years (Nunez, 2021). This increase is attributed to many factors; from improvements in modern medicine to increased access to healthcare and better nutrition and hygiene. Such factors provide our bodies with the ability to protect their cells better, decreasing the amount of damage our cells will experience over the years as we age; thus, improving our life expectancy. So while aging may be inevitable, you *can* slow it down. Numerous methods exist for slowing down the aging process. I will discuss these methods in great detail in the chapters that follow; however, the list below provides you with a brief overview of some of the more important methods you can use to take better care of your body and mind, protect your cells, and increase your life expectancy by slowing down the aging process.

- **Nutritious diet:** It's important that you eat right and try to limit the amount of processed foods you eat where possible. You may need the assistance of a qualified dietician; however, introducing a nutritious diet into your lifestyle involves increasing the number of proteins, whole grains, fruits, and vegetables that you eat.

- **Exercise:** Ideally, an adult should exercise for thirty minutes per day for five days per week. The type of exercise that you do will depend on what you enjoy, but as long as it gets your body moving and stimulates your brain, it will fulfill its role in reducing the mental and physical effects of aging. Such exercises could include yoga, walking, swimming (this type of exercise is great if you have joint issues, past injuries, or arthritis), or even riding your bike.
- **Reduce or avoid tobacco:** Tobacco can have detrimental effects on your health and may contribute to speeding up the aging process. If you are looking to decrease, or completely eliminate, tobacco from your life, it may be worthwhile to seek out the assistance of your local healthcare practitioner. They will be able to guide you on this journey, as well as support you as you face the challenges that often accompany quitting an addictive substance.
- **Limit your alcohol intake:** While enjoying a glass of whiskey or wine every now and then is

okay; if not drunk in moderation, alcohol can increase your chances of developing a chronic disease. According to the Centers for Disease Control and Prevention (CDC) (2022), two drinks per day for men and one drink per day for women is the safest recommended amount of alcohol for those who do choose to drink.

- **Regular checkups:** As we get older, it's normal for illnesses to start developing. As such, I would recommend regularly visiting your local healthcare provider for a routine checkup so that any illnesses can be identified and treated at an early stage. This is especially important if your family has a history of health issues like Alzheimer's or cancer. If your healthcare practitioner is aware of these conditions, they can ensure that the necessary tests and precautions are taken to identify and treat these conditions before they begin. This will also ensure that you take care of your health in a way that is appropriate for these conditions.
- **Stimulate your brain:** Just like you need to exercise your body, you also need to ensure your brain is being regularly stimulated. Solve problems, play games, learn new skills, or do activities that get your brain working. It also

works as a great excuse to try new things and find out what you do and don't like.
- **Sunscreen:** It's important that you protect your skin. Your skin is made up of cells that need to be protected. Products like sunscreen are important for protecting your skin from ultraviolet radiation (UV), especially if you enjoy going out into the sun or taking part in outdoor activities. Additionally, drinking water and skin care products—like moisturizer—should also be used to keep your skin hydrated.

Please note: A person's body requires different amounts and types of things in order to thrive. The above list provides you with a basic overview of the habits that are often used by SuperAgers, but it isn't guaranteed to increase your life expectancy.

THEORIES OF AGING

Now that you understand that you have the ability to influence your life expectancy to a certain degree, you need to understand that there are a multitude of aging theories based on the two different types of aging that affect your body. Cellular aging and damage-related environmental aging are experienced by everyone;

however, how you experience them will differ depending on various factors. This impacts *how* you age and *experience* the aging process. I have briefly explained the two different types of aging below so that you have a better understanding of how the cells in your body are affected as you get older before moving on to the theories of aging.

Two Types of Aging

There are two main types of aging that are affected by factors both inside and outside of your body.

Cellular Aging

Cellular aging is the process by which your cells undergo aging. You cannot actively control this process, as the biological aging of cells is controlled by processes that are normally determined by your genetics. It's a natural process that can be influenced—to a certain degree—by how you take care of your body, but it cannot be controlled. In general, cells will divide and multiply as needed to perform basic biological functions, but the more that they divide, the faster they will age. Eventually, a cell can lose its ability to function properly, resulting in what is known as *cellular damage.* As your body's cells get older, cellular damage increases and starts to negatively affect your overall health. Your body's biological processes may begin to fail as cellular damage accumulates over time.

Damage-Related Environmental Aging

Aging doesn't solely occur inside the body. Factors outside your body also impact how you age. Oftentimes, you have control over these external factors, as they include the environment where you live, your daily habits, and even your stress levels (I will discuss stress management in chapter five). Air pollution, UV radiation, nutrition, and alcohol consumption are additional external factors that influence how your body ages. One-time exposure often won't have a large impact on your health, but the more you are exposed to these factors, the more that the damage caused accumulates, influencing how you age.

Types of Aging Theories

Aging is constantly being studied by the scientific community. As a result, a number of theories exist that can be used to explain the aging process; however, you need to keep in mind that many of these theories are often used in tandem to explain how aging works because many of them overlap with each other.

According to Nunez (2021), the theories below are the five most popular theories that are used to understand how and why aging occurs.

Please note: Many of these theories are still being investigated, with new information and research becoming available to us as technology and science improve.

Genetic Theories

According to this theory, how you age is primarily dependent on your genetics. Genes determine the characteristics that you will inherit from your parents and are found in your chromosomes. Therefore, genes have the ability to influence your life expectancy. Unfortunately, this theory does not account for the influence of external factors on the aging process. It has been estimated that at least 25% of your lifespan is influenced by your genetics (Nunez, 2021). Genetic theories are split up into four additional theories, including the

- **Telomere theory:** The ends of your chromosomes are protected by telomeres. As your chromosomes undergo cell division, these telomeres start shortening. This triggers the aging process and can result in illness (Nunez, 2021).

- **Longevity theory:** It is believed that our genes may have the ability to extend our lifespan (Nunez, 2021). However, research is still being conducted.
- **Stem cell theory:** Stem cells are cells without any particular function that have the ability to form the cells needed to repair tissues and organs in the body. This theory states that as the ability of stem cells starts to decrease over time, the human body will begin aging (Nunez, 2021).
- **Programmed senescence theory:** The process whereby cells that are no longer capable of dividing or growing—but remain alive—is known as *senescence*. The programmed theory of senescence explains how this process is determined by your genetics and acts as an evolutionary tool, influencing how you age (Nunez, 2021).

Evolutionary Theories

You have probably heard of "natural selection." This is when you have certain characteristics or traits that have the ability to help your body adapt to its environment, increasing your chances of survival. Evolutionary theories are based on the idea that the aging process is dependent on natural selection. When you have passed on the traits that have helped you survive to your children, it is believed that you will begin aging; however, this idea is still undergoing research (Nunez, 2021). Currently, three main evolutionary theories exist, including

- **Disposable soma theory:** When you have children, your body will direct its resources towards the reproductive process. This decreases the number of resources needed for DNA repair, resulting in damage to your cells. This damage may be responsible for aging (Nunez, 2021).
- **Antagonistic pleiotropy theory:** It may be possible that the genes that play a role in your fertility have the ability to negatively impact your life at a later stage; therefore, playing a role in the aging process (Nunez, 2021).

Error Theories

Also known as damage theories, they believe that aging is actually caused by random cellular changes (Nunez, 2021). The following six theories make up error theories.

- **Wear and tear theory:** Unfortunately, your cells do experience wear and tear in your body, causing them to break down and become damaged over time. However, this theory ignores the fact that the human body does have the ability to repair itself if properly cared for (Nunez, 2021).

- **Cross-linkage theory:** When two or more proteins become linked together, they are called "cross-linked proteins." Over time, the number of cross-linked proteins build up in your body, damaging your cells and slowing down your body's biological functions, leading to aging (Nunez, 2021).
- **Genome instability theory:** This theory is quite simple and believes that when your body loses its ability to repair any damage to your DNA, you will start to age (Nunez, 2021).
- **Rate-of-living theory:** Your cells' ability to undergo chemical changes to provide energy to your body—known as your *metabolism*—is believed to play a role in determining your life expectancy (Nunez, 2021).
- **Free radical theory:** When there is a disturbance in the balance of free radicals (reactive atoms found in your body that have been introduced through sources such as toxins, tobacco, and smoke) in your body, the aging process will be triggered (Nunez, 2021).

- **Mitochondrial theory:** This theory is a variation of the above theory and believes that damage to your body's mitochondria (organelles that provide energy to your body's cells) can release the free radicals that play a role in aging (Nunez, 2021).

Programmed Theories

While also known as adaptive or aging theories, they are based on the idea that your body has been designed to age (Nunez, 2021). In other words, the life expectancy of your cells has been programmed into your body, and you don't have control over it. The three theories that follow expand more on the idea that we have been designed to age.

- **Gene theory:** This theory suggests that certain genes in your body have the ability to become active or inactive—depending on a variety of factors—causing you to age (Nunez, 2021).
- **Immunological theory:** Otherwise known as the autoimmune theory, it has been suggested that as your immune response declines over time, you will be put at risk for disease and start aging (Nunez, 2021).
- **Endocrine theory:** Your endocrine system consists of glands with the ability to produce

hormones that play a role in your cell's and body's metabolism. When these hormones undergo changes, it's believed that you start to age (Nunez, 2021).

- **Why women often live longer than men:** In many parts of the world, women often live longer than men (Nunez, 2021). This may be due to a variety of reasons such as biological, social, or environmental factors. Women also produce higher amounts of estrogen—a female sex hormone that has the ability to promote the body's anti-inflammatory response and boost the immune system—protecting women from certain diseases (Nunez, 2021). Meanwhile, the male sex hormone—testosterone—can suppresses the immune system. Additionally, men and women practice different behaviors in daily life that can impact their health and, therefore, how they age.

Biochemical Theories

These theories are based on the idea that when a chemical reaction occurs inside of your body—known as a *biochemical reaction*—you will start to age (Nunez, 2021). These reactions are normal and occur throughout your life; however, they are based on various ideas. The three following theories make up the main biochemical theories.

- **Damage accumulation theory:** Your DNA, metabolism, and proteins can become damaged over time when chemical reactions naturally occur in your body (Nunez, 2021).
- **Advanced glycation products (AGEs) theory:** When your body's fats and proteins are exposed to factors such as increased levels of stress and sugars, AGEs begin to develop. This causes an imbalance between your body's free radicals and antioxidant defenses—also called *oxidative stress*—causing you to age faster (Nunez, 2021).
- **Heatshock response theory:** Your cells are protected from stress by heat shock proteins; however, their ability to protect your cells decreases as you get older, leaving your cells more vulnerable as you get older and contributing to the aging process (Nunez, 2021).

METHODS FOR SLOWING DOWN THE AGING PROCESS

Now that you have a basic understanding of the various aging theories that exist, you are probably wondering what you can do to slow down the aging process. The six main anti-aging methods will be explained in more detail in the chapters that follow. However, the section below provides you with a brief sneak peek of what's to come:

- **Positivity:** Positive psychology plays an important role in aging. By learning how to think more positively, you can help your brain thrive. Positivity helps make your daily life appear and feel more enjoyable, helping you look forward to waking up and starting each day. This impacts your attitude about life as you start to develop a more positive outlook.
- **Supplements:** There are a variety of supplements that you can use to help you slow down the aging process. But there are numerous anti-aging supplements on the market, and not all of them do what they promise. You will learn about the supplements that can help you slow down the aging process, as well as how to take them safely, in chapter three.
- **Neuroplasticity:** Your brain's health is important. While positivity plays a role here too, you will learn about neuroplasticity—which is your brain's ability to continuously

grow and evolve as you get older, learn, and experience new things—and how it works and benefits you, as well as how you can improve your brain's capacity for neuroplasticity.

- **Stress management**: Stress can influence how you age, so it's important to learn how to effectively manage your stress, understand the difference between good and bad stress, as well as how exercise and methods like mindfulness are great stress management techniques.
- **Earthing:** This strategy is used to help you connect to the Earth's electric field and decrease the production of free radicals that are harmful to your body. You essentially connect to the Earth to heal your body. Here you will learn about the benefits and types of earthing, as well as its importance and anti-aging effects.
- **Meaningful connections:** Your relationships with others are important. While you don't have to be social all the time, it's important that you learn how to cultivate and nurture meaningful relationships with other people. Here I will expand on the benefits of meaningful connections in the anti-aging process and how to build and maintain these connections throughout your life, in a way that works for you.

KEY TAKEAWAYS

- Aging may be inevitable, but you can use a variety of methods to slow it down.
- Various strategies exist for improving your life expectancy, but they mainly involve taking care of your mental and physical health and allowing yourself to enjoy your life.
- Two main types of aging exist: cellular aging and damage-related environmental aging.
- The two types of aging often occur simultaneously and are affected by factors in your external and internal environment.
- A multitude of theories exists to explain *how* and *why* aging occurs.
- Many of these theories are still being studied, with new information being discovered as technology and science develop.
- There are six main anti-aging methods.

Getting older may not sound appealing, but it's actually an exciting time in your life. You now have the experience and knowledge that you didn't have 20-years ago that you can use to enjoy yourself and live the life you have always dreamed of. This chapter provided you with important information that helped you gain a better understanding of *why* we will be using the specific methods in the chapters that follow to slow down the aging process. It will take time and patience, but don't stop thinking about the benefits you can receive and experience. After all, a positive attitude can take you a long way on your journey toward anti-aging.

2

THE POWER OF A POSITIVE ATTITUDE

> *Never lose the sense of optimism you had as a youth, it'll help keep you young.*
>
> — DAVID D MCCRAY

When you are a teenager, getting older is framed as a good thing. As soon as you hit your twenties, though, society starts telling you that aging means you will become fragile, senile, and unable to actively take part in society. As such, anti-aging products that focus on getting rid of wrinkles and workouts that are supposed to keep your body young are marketed to you—regardless of whether they work or not. With all these "anti-aging" products for sale, it's no wonder many of us feel like getting older is a bad thing.

The negative mindset that it creates can be extremely harmful, especially if you feel a lot younger than your actual age. One important technique for anti-aging that works is a **positive attitude**. When you think of getting older as a bad thing, you probably dread your birthdays —feeling sad and depressed when you realize that you're an entire year older. However, when you think about aging in a more positive light—one where getting older means you can now take part in activities that need more experience and wisdom that can only be achieved with getting older—you start to feel excited about your birthdays, and look forward to the adventures and opportunities that the new year will bring. When you look at aging from these two different perspectives, you realize that age really is a meaningless number and that having a positive mindset is important for helping you thrive.

THE BRAIN THRIVES ON POSITIVITY

Before we move on to *why* the brain thrives on positivity, you first need to have a basic understanding of *how* your brain functions. The part of the brain that regulates and responds to emotions—both positive and negative emotions—is known as the *amygdala*. When a person uses positivity to improve their attitude towards life, their brain's chemistry changes. Brain chemistry can influence whether you feel positively or negatively about a situation or person. According to Achieve Medical Center (2020), positive thinking has been associated with an increase in cells in the human body that have the ability to improve the immune system, thereby protecting the body and mind from harmful external influences.

Positive emotions also impact the part of your brain known as the *prefrontal cortex*. This part of your brain is essential to the connection between your mind and body. If you need to find specific information, your prefrontal cortex is the one that searches for it. Your neurons—also known as signals because of their ability to look for information—provide the prefrontal cortex with the information they found, allowing you the opportunity to evaluate it. The areas that connect your neurons, called *synapses,* increase when you develop a positive attitude. This can help you improve your ability to control and regulate your emotions, focus better, solve problems, and identify how you think, while also improving your creative thinking ability, attention span, and intellectual adaptability.

Generated by your brain's neurons, positivity encourages the production of serotonin in your brain. Serotonin is a hormone that plays an important role in mood regulation and memory function. Simply put, when your brain produces serotonin, you feel good about yourself and your life. You find it easier to stay positive about your life as you get older. As such, properly regulated serotonin levels will allow you to remain emotionally stable, feel less anxious, improve your focus, and feel calmer and happier overall.

But it's unrealistic to think that you can have a positive attitude *all* the time. You are only human, and it's normal to experience a variety of emotions, even negative ones. While negative thinking isn't ideal, it's normal to have days where you feel sad, tired, or stressed out. What matters is that you don't get stuck in these emotions because they can affect your mind and body. Remember that your emotions are impacted by your environment, so don't be afraid to make changes that could improve your attitude about a situation. If you get stuck in your negative thoughts and feelings, you may find it difficult to solve problems, think creatively or experience new ideas, control your impulses, or feel good about something that would normally bring a smile to your face. Don't worry, you can learn how to intentionally shift your negative mood and attitude to a more positive way of thinking that will be beneficial to your health and well-being.

The Power of a Positive Attitude

You may be able to improve your health by developing a positive attitude. According to Harvard T.H. Chan School of Public Health (2022), in a study of 14,000 adults over 50-years-old, 43% had a lower risk of dying from any cause over a 4-year-period. This means that a positive attitude about getting older may help you live a longer, healthier life. The study also found that individuals with a more positive attitude had a lower risk of diabetes, stroke, cancer, and heart disease; as well as better cognitive functioning. They were also more likely to exercise, had less trouble sleeping, experienced less loneliness and depression, and were more optimistic, with a greater sense of purpose (Harvard T.H. Chan School of Public Health, 2022).

This study shows you that you don't have to give in to society's belief that getting older means you need to become frail, cranky, or lament your so-called "lost youth." Recognize your own accomplishments and contributions to your life, despite your age. A positive attitude is merely there to reinforce your sense of purpose and happiness, allowing you to remain a competent individual who can contribute to their community despite their age. You can start shifting your attitude to one that is more positive by using small steps, but you have to actively work on it every day.

DEVELOPING A POSITIVE ATTITUDE

You have probably realized by now that your mind is pretty powerful if you understand it and actively work to utilize its power. This is important for improving your attitude towards life and getting older. You need to remember, however, that on your journey to anti-aging, you won't be perfect, and you don't have to be. You can still be proud of your accomplishments and successes, even if they're small. What's important is that you embrace taking responsibility for your thoughts, actions, and feelings when you do make mistakes during this process. This will help you cultivate a sense of respect for not only yourself, but also the people in your life and environment. Before I move on to *why* a positive attitude can benefit you, I want you to answer the following questions so that you can determine whether your attitude is currently more negative or positive.

- Reflect on your relationships with the people in your life. Are these relationships beneficial to your well-being?
- Is the environment in which you live (whether it's an apartment, house, or simply a room you frequent) positive? In other words, does it inspire positive feelings? Or do you feel sad and depressed when you are here?
- What changes can you make to your environment to improve it and make it more positive? These changes should make you happy. Don't listen to others if they say that a change is childish or unfashionable—like decorating your couch with pillows shaped like ghosts because you like Halloween, or painting your bedroom dark green because it's your favorite color.
- Using your daily routine, identify whether it helps you feel positive about yourself and your life?
- Are you able to identify your state of mind in the present moment?

- Can you actively notice when your state of mind changes?

Use your answers to these questions to help you identify *how* you can make getting older more enjoyable. This often involves introducing things into your living space that make you happy, or even changing your appearance in some way—like dying your hair—because no one can tell you not to. This is your life. You may be getting older but that doesn't mean you can't enjoy yourself. If anything, allowing yourself to live your life the way you want to will not only make you happier and improve your attitude towards aging, but it will also inspire those younger than you to start enjoying their lives.

Benefits of a Positive Attitude

Throughout this chapter, I briefly mentioned all the different ways a positive attitude about aging can be beneficial. However, there are additional benefits to actively improving your attitude towards getting older. These benefits are briefly mentioned below.

A Happier Life

While life is unpredictable, and certainly not perfect, you have the power to make it enjoyable. A positive attitude helps you see a negative situation in a way that creates opportunities for you instead of becoming another problem to solve. This can help you bring out your best qualities and start enjoying your life.

Health Benefits

I briefly mentioned the benefits of a positive attitude on your health earlier in this chapter. In addition to what was previously mentioned, when you actively try to maintain a positive attitude towards aging, you may be able to boost your immune system, strengthen your body, improve your illness recovery time, and reduce your risk of a heart attack. Mentally, you start becoming more alert and lower your risk of mental health issues. You might also live longer if you enjoy your life and see getting older as a fun and educational adventure.

Success

When you look at your life in a more positive light, you may have a greater chance of being successful because you aren't focusing on "what ifs" or what could go wrong. You may also feel more inspired to start a new day and face the challenges that pursuing success can bring.

Increased Energy

A positive attitude can increase your energy levels because you feel excited about your life, helping you achieve more every day. You can channel your positivity into your work (if you have not yet retired), hobbies, volunteer work, relationships, or things that you enjoy doing every day—like gardening, painting, or even knitting. This may improve your focus and help you cultivate your enthusiasm.

Positivity itself has a great many benefits regardless of your age, gender, and whether you are retired or are still working. While it's important to understand how a positive attitude can benefit you as you get older, how exactly do you develop a positive attitude?

How to Develop a Positive Attitude

There are a multitude of ways to cultivate a positive attitude. While this section is not a comprehensive list, I have included the most popular and frequently used strategies for changing your attitude towards life and aging. You will need to go through each strategy and determine whether it will work for you or not. I would suggest trying each technique a few times before moving on to a new strategy—or even combining them —as it does take time before you will start experiencing any results. Patience and consistency is key to developing a positive attitude. Don't be hard on yourself when you make mistakes or struggle to implement a technique. The methods below are some of the strategies that you can use to improve your attitude towards getting older, as well as towards your daily life.

Listen to Yourself

The little voice in our heads is with us 24/7. You have to notice how this voice talks about you, as self-talk can impact your self-esteem and confidence. If it's constantly negative and criticizing you, then you will struggle to see the good in daily life or feel positive emotions about yourself. Many of our voices start out as negative because of society's influence as we grow up. It says that you shouldn't do this specific thing because you are too "old," but in reality, you feel like you're only 20-years-old. Or it tells you that you should be sitting at home, wasting away in front of your television because you are now retired. But just because that little voice believes it right doesn't mean it is. You need to actively notice how this voice speaks to you and work on changing its attitude to one that is more positive using methods like affirmations, mindfulness, or even gratitude journaling.

Interact With Positive People and Environments

Taking note of your inner dialogue is important, but you also have to determine whether your environment and even the people you spend your time with, have negative or positive attitudes. Your attitude will be influenced the more time you spend with someone or in a specific place. Take the time to go to places that hold special meaning or memories for you. The people you spend your time with should also positively affect you, instead of making you feel bad about yourself or your age. It's your life, and you deserve better than people who hurt you or make you feel bad about yourself.

Volunteer

If you are looking to ensure that your life gives you a sense of fulfillment or purpose as you get older, you could partake in activities like volunteering. It not only gives you a reason to wake up every day, but it also keeps your mind and body busy, as well as helping you contribute to the community. Spending time with others who are trying to make a difference will help you realize that there is still good in the world—which is a great way to reinforce a positive attitude.

Laugh

Laughter has been compared to medicine for many years, and there is a valid reason behind this. It acts as a mood enhancer by releasing endorphins into your body, decreasing your stress levels, reducing tension, and making it easier for you to cope during stressful and difficult situations. You don't need something big to make you laugh. Laugh at the little things in your life; if you mess something up or even make a fool of yourself by walking into a wall, laugh at yourself! Everyone makes stupid mistakes and acts goofy when they are left alone. Being able to accept this side of yourself and allowing yourself to laugh can make you happier and change your attitude for the better.

Love Yourself and Allow Others to Love You

As you get older, you need to accept yourself for who you are despite your flaws, mistakes, and age. Accepting yourself for who you are is important as you go on the journey to anti-aging. The one message that I keep reinforcing is that your age is merely a number. It doesn't determine how old you feel on the inside or whether you will enjoy your life. You deserve to experience love, even if you are the one providing it. Sometimes, embracing self-love can be the most important step to accepting yourself for who you are and enjoying your life.

Take Care of Yourself

Self-love and self-care often go hand-in-hand. The ultimate act of self-love is actively taking care of yourself and attending to **your** needs and wants. Physical and mental health is important, especially as you get older. You may feel as young as 20, but your body often needs special attention and care, too. Everyone has experienced life differently; as such, you may have old injuries or new ones—like arthritis—that start impacting your body and mind. You need to make sure that you always pay attention to your mind and body and attend to their needs.

Self-care is a daily practice that allows you to take a moment to step back from your daily life and breathe, helping you relax and purposefully take time for yourself. It takes on many forms and includes the following behaviors: Watching a movie, getting takeout, reading, doing skincare (skin care is important for both men and women regardless of their age), baking, eating your favorite dessert, or even just saying "no" to plans that others have made so that you can do what *you* want.

Take a Break!

Breaks are important. It doesn't matter whether or not you have already retired. You should take at least 30-minutes a day for yourself. Step away from your workspace or the environment you've been spending time in. Go and have lunch or a snack, take a nap, walk around the block, or do something for yourself. Actively taking time to rest every day will help you feel motivated and re-energized. Additionally, you will also find it easier to keep a positive attitude throughout your day.

Make Plans for the End of the Day

Taking a few nights every week to plan something that you enjoy—going out for dinner with friends or family, watching your favorite movie, or having a night in—can give you something to look forward to at the end of your day, helping you stay positive, and motivating you to continue with your day. Remember, it doesn't matter whether you have retired yet or not, it's good to get out and do things for yourself because it helps you maintain balance in your life, have fun, and take time to focus on yourself.

Listen to Music

Listen to music that matches your current mood. This will look different for everyone because we all have different music tastes. Occasionally, a person may listen to sad music to feel happy because the beauty and emotions in the music makes them feel good; while others need to listen to an upbeat, exciting song that gets their blood pumping and allows them to dance around their house. Even if you feel ridiculous while doing it–you must enjoy yourself. Feeling slightly silly every now and then doesn't really matter when you feel motivated to carry on with your life and pursue each day with renewed energy and a sense of purpose.

You don't need to have a specific purpose in life—like doctors who save lives or life coaches who help others find themselves—sometimes life's purpose can merely be about enjoying it. As you get older, I think it's more important that you are enjoying your life than conforming to society's stereotypes or allowing others to make you feel bad about wanting to change your life. Embrace the age that you feel and live your life how **you** want to live.

POSITIVE THINKING EXERCISE

Using the contents of this chapter, I want you to use the activities that follow to help you change your attitude towards life. You can practice these activities one at a time, or you can even combine them to create an activity that suits you and your lifestyle better. As you saw above, a multitude of positive thinking exercises exist; however, the methods below are the most commonly used methods for changing your attitude to one that is more positive.

Believe in Yourself

You need to appreciate yourself for who you are. This is practiced through activities like self-care (which I mentioned above). Stand in front of your mirror and say, out loud, what you like about yourself, your life, and anything else that you think is important. You should also praise yourself and your accomplishments —even if they're small. For example, you could say, "I am a wonderful person and my age doesn't determine my self-worth or ability to do the things I love."

Positive Affirmations

Affirmations are a great way to improve your attitude and help you become more optimistic about life. The more you repeat positive affirmations, the more effective they'll become. You can also practice your affirmations in front of the mirror to help you reinforce them. Practice these positive statements every day. They can help you feel good about yourself mentally and physically. As such, the statements that you use should carry a special meaning for you. You can either create your own affirmations or use statements from the internet that speak to you. Positive affirmations include ones like the following:

- I am worth the effort.
- My age doesn't determine my worth or ability to enjoy life.
- I am proud of myself for getting up each day to live my life to the fullest, even if that's simply taking care of my garden.
- What I do matters.

Embrace the Present

Stop dwelling on the past and the future. You are here in the present, so live in it! The past can't be changed—well, unless you have a time machine, but science has not yet invented those. Work on bringing your attention to the present and live your life in the now. Find activities that keep your attention focused on the present moment—like volunteering, spending time with family or friends, or even participating in one of your hobbies.

Breathe

Breathing can help you bring your attention to the present by focusing on it. Take a deep breath and pretend you are breathing out the negative emotions that are affecting you. Focus on your breath so that you can clear your mind and think about the current situation in a more rational manner. This will help you make the best decision in a difficult situation and help you remain in the present.

Be Kind to Yourself

Stop judging yourself for your mistakes. We are all constantly learning, even as we get older. But fear of failure can prevent us from living the life we want, especially as we get older. Instead of judging yourself for your behavior or mistakes, try to find the opportunity that failure brings you and figure out how you can use it to your advantage. Being kind to yourself is about forgiving yourself, being patient and sympathetic towards yourself, and allowing yourself to be who you truly are without judgment—even if that's a 10-year-old in the body of an 80-year-old.

Gratitude Journaling

Journaling is a great way to stay positive about your life. It may feel weird or childish, but its benefits and positive impact outweigh feeling a bit silly. Write down three things every day that you are grateful for in a notebook and allow yourself to fully acknowledge them. They can be large—like having a loving family and friends—or small—like treating yourself to your favorite dessert or drink without judgment. What you write down every day is essentially up to you. The key here is that the thing you write down is something good that you can appreciate. Gratitude journaling helps you feel grateful for your current life and find the good in each day, helping you reinforce a positive attitude towards your life.

Read an Inspiring Book

It can be difficult to overcome challenges, or even stereotypes, about aging. Don't be afraid to read a book that makes you feel motivated and inspired about pursuing anti-aging methods. That's one of the main purposes of this book. Reading about things that inspire you and make you feel capable of overcoming the challenges in your life will change your attitude towards aging and taking part in activities that bring you happiness for the better.

Use Positive Language

Combine this activity with listening to your inner dialogue. When you talk to yourself, avoid the use of negative words or language like "don't," "can't," or "won't." Notice how you speak to yourself, and actively work on changing it so that the phrasing is more positive and helps you feel better about yourself and more capable. Instead of saying, "I can't learn to ski at 70-years-old," say, "I can learn to ski at 70-years-old because my age is merely a number, and I am capable and enjoy learning new things."

Personal Mantra

Positive language and affirmations can help you create a personal mantra. This mantra is a personal phrase that inspires you and makes you feel more positive about your daily life. Repeat your mantra to yourself every day. You can practice in front of the mirror, or carry this phrase with you on a note card. One example of a possible mantra is, "I am worth the effort I put in, despite the mistakes I have made."

KEY TAKEAWAYS

- Aging has been framed as a bad thing for many years, but that doesn't mean it is.
- You can overcome this negative mindset towards aging by using positivity.
- Understanding how your brain works will help you improve your attitude by increasing your serotonin production.
- A positive attitude has many benefits. It can help you feel more positively about getting older, allowing you to remain happy even as the years pass by.
- Positivity helps you recognize and celebrate your accomplishments despite your age.

- You have to actively work to take notice of your attitude towards aging and how society's stereotypes impact you in order to change your attitude to one that is more positive.

You can't be positive all the time; you are only human, after all. A positive attitude towards aging is important for enjoying the rest of your life and feeling good about yourself despite your age. Additionally, positivity can impact your physical and mental health, but sometimes you may need extra help. Chapter three focuses on the different supplements that you can use to take care of and improve your mental and physical health as you get older.

SHARING THE SECRETS OF THE SUPER AGERS

> *"Knowledge is power. Sharing knowledge is the key to unlocking that power."*
>
> — MARTIN UZOCHUKWU UGWU

As you learn the secrets of the super agers and begin to change your life according to their methods, you may find yourself becoming increasingly aware of the deteriorating health of older people around you.

The very reason you chose to pick up this book and begin taking steps to reverse the effects of aging is undoubtedly likely to spark concern for those around you and make you wish more people had the insights necessary to reset their biological clocks and live healthy and vibrant lives long into old age.

It wouldn't surprise me at all if you've already shared some of what you've learned with your friends and family members... But what if I told you that you could help me spread the word even further?

It might surprise you to learn just how simple it is to do that.

By leaving a review of this book on Amazon, you can help other readers find the information they need that you're already beginning to see transform your life.

By spending just a few minutes to review this book, you can let other people know how it has helped you and what they'll find inside. Simply by doing that, you'll let new readers know that this is the book they're looking for, and, together, we'll be able to spread the word even further. Who knows... Collectively, we could end up pushing the life expectancy figure up even further!

Thank you so much for helping me spread the word. If we're going to live longer, we want to make sure we're healthy and well through all the years we have left in front of us – and you're helping me make that possible for even more people.

Scan the QR code below for a quick review!

3

AGE-DEFYING SUPPLEMENTS

Mentally, you may feel years younger than your true age, but your body probably didn't get the same message. As you get older, your body experiences what is known as *cellular senescence,* which I discussed briefly in Chapter 1. Remember that *senescence* is when your body's cells lose their ability to divide and grow, but they remain alive in your body. As the years go by, the number of senescent cells builds up, and they begin affecting the aging process and even age-related diseases. But everyone ages at a different rate. This is due to a variety of factors, like your genetics, how you take care of yourself, your environment, and even your exposure to things like free radicals. As such, your body may need a little bit of extra help to cope with the aging process.

WHAT ARE SUPPLEMENTS?

Your body may be affected by the years, but that doesn't mean you have to sit on the sidelines, unable to do anything about it. Introducing things like supplements into your diet can help you provide your body with what it needs to thrive. Supplements are the vitamins and minerals that your body needs but may struggle to produce or absorb on its own from your diet. They are taken in the form of capsules, tablets, injections, or powders. However, age-defying supplements cannot reverse the aging process. They merely help you attend to and meet your body's needs in a way that can improve and maintain your health while also slowing down the effects of aging on both your mind and body.

Dietary Supplements

Supplementing your diet with vitamins and minerals can be quite useful as you get older. They help you add nutrients to your diet in the form of enzymes, amino acids, plants, herbs, vitamins, and minerals. This is especially helpful when you are unable to introduce them through your diet or your body struggles to absorb them from your food. Fortunately, supplements don't require a prescription and are often readily available at your nearest grocery store or pharmacy. It is recommended that individuals over the age of 50-years-old start to introduce supplements into their diet (Mayer Robinson, 2021). As you get older, there are three main supplements that are often recommended for ensuring that your mind and body continue to thrive with a lower risk of issues.

Calcium

This mineral is important for ensuring that your bones stay strong and healthy as you get older. After the age of 50, you begin to lose bone mass—something that is especially common among women—which puts you at risk of fractures or breaking your bones if you fall. Calcium can be found in foods like canned fish, milk, and dark green, leafy vegetables. Take vitamin D with your calcium supplement, as vitamin D helps your body better absorb the calcium (Mayer Robinson, 2021).

Vitamin D

If you need to take a calcium supplement, you should also take a vitamin D supplement, as it will help your body fully absorb the calcium. As you get older, your body may find it difficult to produce enough vitamin D—which can normally be produced after 15 to 30 minutes of exposure to sunlight—so you may have to begin taking a supplement. Additionally, vitamin D can be found in foods like fatty fish, fortified cereal, and fortified milk (Mayer Robinson, 2021).

Vitamin B12

Getting older means learning how to keep track of your body's vitamin and mineral levels, as a deficiency can led to the onset of age-related diseases or simply harm your body and speed up the aging process. Your stomach acid levels will begin to decrease as you get older; as such, your body may begin to struggle absorbing vitamin B12, which is absorbed through stomach acid. This vitamin is vital for preventing anemia by ensuring the health of your red blood cells and nerves. Vitamin B12 can be found in the form of a tablet, an injection, or even in meats and fortified cereals (Mayer Robinson, 2021).

Besides the more common dietary supplements (I have included a brief overview of some of these supplements later in the chapter) that are often recommended, there are two additional types of supplements that each have a different effect on your body and play a different role in combating the aging process. They include antioxidants and herbal supplements.

Antioxidants

Antioxidants may have the ability to slow the onset of age-related diseases. They often include vitamins C and E, beta-carotene, and selenium. You can also introduce antioxidants through your diet by including seafood, seeds, nuts, fruits, and vegetables in your meals (Mayer Robinson, 2021). Remember that the number of antioxidants that you need will differ from the amounts needed by others. As such, please consult your medical practitioner or even a dietician to ensure that you are ingesting the correct number of antioxidants for your body's needs.

Antioxidants: Myths Versus Reality

There are many myths about the anti-aging effects of antioxidants, but what is the truth? First, you need to understand that antioxidants aren't a miracle cure for aging that will somehow rid your body of any and all toxins and make you look 20-years younger. I mentioned free radicals in Chapter 1, and one thing you need to remember is that they have the ability to speed up the aging process. The truth is that antioxidants have the ability to protect your cells from the damage caused to your body and skin that normally results from free radicals.

Many companies sell creams containing antioxidants, claiming they will reverse the damage to your skin cells that causes wrinkles and dark spots. However, antioxidants that are found in topical skin creams only have a short-term effect, and sometimes they don't even make a difference because it's difficult for your skin to absorb antioxidants.

While many myths exist surrounding antioxidants and other anti-aging supplements, you also need to remember that research and clinical studies are constantly being conducted to study the effects of these supplements on your body as well as what formulations will be stable enough to actually be effective. As such, there will always be new research available on the benefits of using antioxidants, as well as their effects.

Herbal Supplements

While herbal supplements can have many benefits for your health as you get older, they also have the ability to interfere with your current medications, supplements, and even existing medical conditions, causing unpleasant side effects. Examples of some popular herbal supplements include ginkgo biloba, black cohosh, ginseng, and echinacea. Before you introduce herbal supplements into your life, please speak with your healthcare provider to ensure that the supplements you would like to take won't interfere with your current medications, supplements, health conditions, or cause adverse effects.

Are Supplements Safe?

Vitamins and minerals in general have a unique effect on different individuals. This is due to the natural occurrence of different levels of these vitamins and minerals in your body and diet. As diets differ between households, you may already be receiving some of these vitamins and minerals from your food. And supplements are exactly that—a supplement to your diet. They provide you with the vitamins and minerals that you aren't getting enough of or that your body struggles to create and absorb. I do recommend that you consult a qualified medical practitioner—and even a dietician—before using any of the supplements mentioned in this chapter. Additionally, please remember that the benefits mentioned in this chapter cannot be guaranteed, as studies, research, and clinical trials are still being conducted on many of these supplements.

Supplements can be safe when taken in the appropriate amount and in a form that your body has no problem absorbing. However, they can also be harmful when taken in high doses or with supplements or medications that could create a dangerous reaction in your body. Additionally, a supplement can be dangerous to take before surgery because of its additional properties. Olive leaf extract, for example, is a supplement often used to boost your immune system, but it's also a blood thinner. As such, it would be dangerous for a person to take this supplement before surgery or if they have a blood-related disorder like hemophilia.

Supplements are often readily available because they are not regulated like over-the-counter medications. This means that their label may make false claims or omit possible side effects and dangers. It's one of the reasons why I keep reiterating that you should consult a qualified medical professional and dietician before introducing supplements, or mineral and vitamin-rich foods into your daily life.

Tips for Taking Supplements

There are five main tips for introducing supplements into your daily life:

- Try the generic version of a supplement, as it is often identical to the name brand version of the same supplement.
- Speak with your local healthcare provider to determine whether the supplement is safe, or

even necessary, for you to take.

- Unless instructed otherwise by a medical professional, ensure that you eat before taking your supplements to prevent an upset stomach and nausea, as well as ensuring that they are absorbed properly.
- Eat as well as you can. If you are unsure about whether your diet is suited to your specific lifestyle and the needs of your body, you can consult your local dietician. Eating well can also help you introduce supplements into your diet in a more natural form if your body does not struggle to absorb them. This includes a variety of fruits and vegetables, lean meats, and whole grains.

TOP FIVE PICKS FOR LONGEVITY

The supplements that I refer to in this section are believed to play a more direct role in influencing your life expectancy. While each supplement has a vast amount of information available on it, I have provided you with a brief overview of the role of each supplement and how it may benefit you. Remember that supplements affect everyone differently. The top five supplements related to influencing your longevity include the following.

Modified Citrus Pectin (MCP)

Found in the peels and pulps of citrus fruits like apples, oranges, and grapefruits, to name a few, this dietary fiber can help you to get rid of the toxic metals that build up over time in your body, prevent diarrhea—especially if you suffer from irritable bowel syndrome (IBS)—slow down the onset of heart disease and cancer growth, as well as improve your brain's health over time. MCP can also be taken in the form of a capsule or powder supplement if you are unable to digest or access citrus fruits.

NAD and Cell Regeneration

As you get older, your stem cells start losing their ability to change into unique cells and multiply as needed. Eventually, this will result in your tissues breaking down and contributing to the aging process. If you introduce a supplement, like a NAD^+-raising compound, you can give these stem cells a new lease on life by extending their lifespan. Essentially, your tissues will be rejuvenated and have the ability to heal your internal and external injuries, ensuring the correct functioning of your body's homeostasis—the process whereby your body's self-regulated internal environment maintains its balance to ensure the internal environment's conditions are suitable for survival. By ensuring your body's cell regeneration is working correctly, your aging process may slow down and delay the onset of age-related illnesses (Wu and Sinclair, 2016).

Ashwagandha

In chapter 1, I mentioned that your mitochondria's telomerase has the ability to limit the number of times your cells can divide. As such, when your cells replicate, your telomeres will ensure that your chromosomes don't fuse together or rearrange, resulting in adverse consequences like cancer. As such, your telomeres may play a role in determining whether you will have a healthy lifespan or not. The Ashwagandha root is an Ayurvedic medicinal herb that can increase your telomerase's activity, possibly playing a role in anti-aging (Raguraman & Subramaniam, 2016). As such, it may have the ability to increase your telomerase's activity, resulting in decreased loss of telomeres and possibly delaying the aging process.

Senolytic Activator

As you get older, your health is affected by your cellular senescence. Your organs and tissues start to develop a buildup of senescent cells, degrading your tissues and putting you at risk of developing age-related diseases and possibly decreasing your lifespan. Senolytic drugs can be used to eliminate this buildup of senescent cells and improve your health.

TA-65

Often found in traditional Chinese medicines, this dietary supplement can activate your mitochondria's telomeres. Activating your telomeres may increase your cells' ability to regenerate, reduce your risk of developing age-related diseases, increase your resistance to infections, and improve your lifespan.

In addition to the above supplements that play a role in improving your longevity, there are a multitude of supplements that can help you improve your overall health, lifespan, and general mental and physical functioning as you get older. These supplements will affect everyone differently, but it's always good to know what's available to you and how it may be able to benefit you.

SUPPLEMENTS LIST

Many of the supplements discussed in this section require the assistance of a qualified medical professional before being introduced into your life. They can help you determine which supplements could benefit you, in what form this supplement is best taken, and the correct dosage that will help your mind and body thrive as you get older. Consulting a qualified medical practitioner will also help you ensure that your supplements don't negatively interact with any medications you may be taking. Use the information in the list that follows to help you determine which supplements may provide you with the benefits that you are looking for.

- **Coenzyme (CoQ10):** When you get older, your body's CoQ10 levels decrease. This antioxidant has the ability to reduce the buildup of free radicals in your body, which often accelerate the aging process. Therefore, CoQ10 can slow down the aging process by reducing the impact of oxidative stress on your body, protecting your cells from damage and even improving the production of energy in your body. Taking a CoQ10 supplement can help you improve your quality of life as you get older, but you should speak with your healthcare provider before pursuing this supplement (Admin, 2020).
- **Curcumin:** This antioxidant is found in turmeric, a common spice that can be bought at your grocery store. Curcumin has the ability to

activate proteins—like sirtuins and AMP-activated protein kinase (AMPK)—that can delay cellular senescence. As such, this antioxidant may be able to combat damage to your cells, postpone the onset of age-related diseases, and it has anti-inflammatory properties that are beneficial if you struggle with arthritis and joint pain. Curcumin is also beneficial in delaying aging in the brain. You can either take a curcumin supplement or use turmeric in your cooking (Admin, 2020).

- **B12:** This vitamin has the ability to improve the quality and growth of your skin, hair, and nails, whose quality normally declines as you get older. Additionally, it can help you reduce the severity of any mental health issues, as it boosts your energy levels and helps you maintain a positive attitude. B12 is useful for those who would like to maintain a consistent weight and increase their metabolism and appetite, while also protecting against the onset of age-related brain disorders. You can find this vitamin as a supplement, receive it through an injection, or ingest it through your diet. Foods containing B12 include animal products (meats, seafood, and dairy), breakfast cereals, and protein bars (Invigor Medical, 2020).

- **Folic acid**: Also known as vitamin B9 or vitamin M, folic acid is naturally found in broccoli, lentils, asparagus, beans, and leafy, green vegetables, strawberries, peanuts, liver, and orange juice. You can also apply it topically to your skin in the form of a cream containing folic acid. Folic acid plays an important role in the repair, growth, and development of your skin cells. It also slows down premature skin aging by stimulating and promoting red blood cell production and working to maintain the health of your central nervous system. Folic acid can also prevent damage to your DNA (DSM, n.d.).
- **AMPK:** This molecule can help you control the regulation of your body's internal environment to ensure it remains stable so that your cells are able to survive and thrive. As such, it plays a role in the growth and death of your body's cells (which affect how you age, as well as your longevity), and helps you maintain your metabolism. When activated, AMPK can protect your body against cellular senescence, improving your lifespan. Resveratrol, metformin, and exercise are the three main examples being studied in relation to the activation of the AMPK necessary for slowing

down the aging process, but AMPK can be bought in the form of tablet supplements (Stancu, 2015).

- **Magnesium**: As you get older, it's normal for your magnesium levels to decrease; however, low magnesium levels have also been linked to age-related diseases and the acceleration of cellular senescence of your skin cells. As such, a magnesium supplement can help you prevent, or delay, the onset of age-related diseases (Killilea and Maier, 2008).
- **Vitamin K with calcium:** This supplement protects your body against oxidative stress and takes on the role of protector by acting as an anti-inflammatory (Simes et al., 2019).
- **Carditone:** A herbal product that you can use to maintain your blood pressure and reduce your cholesterol levels. Its ability to remain in your bloodstream for a while means you only need to take one dose per day; however, please seek guidance from your medical provider to ensure it won't interfere with any medication you are currently taking, especially for your blood pressure and cholesterol (MedFriendly, 2019)
- **Zinc:** When your body ages, your cells go through complex processes. Even your immune

system undergoes changes, but they can also compromise it. Low levels of zinc are common in aging individuals, but they can cause your immune system to age faster and result in an oxidative inflammatory response that damages your body's cells. By taking a supplement—with zinc being an essential micronutrient—you can boost your immune system, helping it function effectively (Cabrera, 2015).

- **Quercetin:** An antioxidant that can be used to slow down the aging process by directly reducing your body's levels of oxidative stress. Additionally, it is thought that quercetin may be able to resolve the damage caused by cellular senescence in your mind and body (Sohn et al., 2018).
- **Vitamin D:** You may be able to regulate the rate at which you age by taking a vitamin D supplement, which can delay the onset of age-related diseases. This vitamin may also be able to improve and maintain the processes that drive the aging process—such as mitochondrial dysfunction, inflammation, and oxidative stress (Berridge, 2017).
- **Vitamin C:** Your skin is one of the largest organs and suffers the most from exposure to environmental stressors. The antioxidants

found in vitamin C can be used to help protect your skin by defending against UV radiation damage, lightening dark patches of skin, and reduce wrinkles and fine lines when used as a topical cream for more than two weeks. Vitamin C encourages the production of collagen, protecting your body's proteins from being damaged and making it easier for your wounds to heal. Additionally, you can use vitamin C to help repair the damage caused by free radicals, preventing damaged cells from becoming cancerous and slowing down the aging process. Eating right is important and this vitamin can be found in foods like broccoli, red peppers, spinach, and citrus fruits (WebMD Editorial Contributors & Vogin, 2002).

- **Vitamin A:** Found in animal products (meat, poultry, and dairy) and plant products (vegetables and fruits), this vitamin can be used to support the health of your skin, eyes, reproductive health, and immune function. You can also use it to reduce wrinkles and fine lines by applying vitamin A in the form of a topical cream. This vitamin can also improve your skin's elasticity, reduce damage to your cells, and delay the onset of disease (Whelan and Santos-Longhurst, 2022).

- **Vitamin E:** Often considered an important antioxidant, this vitamin can be used to protect your cell membranes and prevent damage to the enzymes associated with your cells. It may also help deactivate free radicals—reducing the amount of damage they can cause—as well as limit the production of cancer cells when applied to your skin in the form of a topical cream. Vitamin E can be found in vegetable oils, dairy products, grains, nuts, and oats (WebMD Editorial Contributors and Vogin, 2002).
- **Taurine:** You can use this antioxidant to help you control the effects of oxidative stress on your body, possibly reducing their impact on the aging process. Taurine is important for the healthy functioning of your brain as you get older due to its anti-inflammatory and antioxidant properties. You can take a taurine tablet supplement or eat beef, poultry, and fish (Codiva, 2022).
- **Lithium:** Lithium may have the ability to slow down the molecular aging process in your cells, but the results depend on your genetics. High levels of lithium in the water have been linked to a longer life expectancy and reduced risk of neurodegenerative diseases (King's College London, 2017). Lithium can also restore your

telomeres and prevent premature cell aging, but require the assistance of a qualified medical professional to determine if it will work for you (King's College London, 2017).

- **Melatonin:** An antioxidant hormone that reduces the damage to oxidative stress and regulates senescence caused by exposure to radiation (like sun exposure). Normally used to help a person sleep, it can help improve hyperpigmentation, heal cell damage, and reduce inflammation.
- **Glutathione:** Found in nearly every cell in your body, this antioxidant plays a role in detoxification (a process that gets rid of toxic substances from your body). It can also lighten dark skin patches, reduce wrinkles, and increase your skin's elasticity (Weshawal et al., 2017).
- **Omega fatty acids:** Omega-3 fatty acids act as an anti-inflammatory that can reduce joint pain and neutralize the free radicals that contribute to your skin's aging process. You can also use it to improve your memory and cognitive functioning. Additionally, omega-3 fatty acids have the ability to act as an antidepressant by boosting your mood, reducing oxidative stress, and lowering your risk of heart disease, type 2

diabetes, arthritis, and Alzheimer's. They are normally found in salmon, chia seeds, flaxseed oil, fish oil, green plants, and grass-fed meat products (Kelly, 2017).

- **Selenium:** A mineral that protects the body from cancer (skin cancer is often caused by excessive sun exposure), preserves your tissue elasticity, and slows down tissue's aging. It can provide protection against UV damage and is found in whole grain cereals, seafood, garlic, and eggs, or you can take it as an oral supplement (WebMD Editorial Contributors and Vogin 2002).

KEY TAKEAWAYS

- Mentally, you may not feel very old, but that doesn't mean your body isn't affected by the aging process.
- You can introduce supplements into your diet to provide your body with the vitamins and minerals it needs to thrive.
- Supplements don't reverse the aging process, but they can delay—or even prevent—the onset of many age-related diseases.
- You can take supplements in the form of a tablet, capsule, powder, injection, or even

introduce foods that contain a high level vitamins or minerals.

- Supplements have both advantages and disadvantages. As such, you should speak with your medical provider before taking a specific, or even combination of, supplements.
- There are a variety of supplements that can benefit you as you get older.

While I haven't mentioned specific brands of supplements, the information that you have been provided with in this chapter will help you make a more informed decision about whether you should personally take supplements, how to introduce them, and what supplements may be beneficial for you. Remember that they are often easy to access, but they aren't regulated like over-the-counter medications, so you will need to be cautious of what the labels on a supplement claim. Now that you understand how you can provide your mind and body with the nutrients, vitamins, and minerals that they need to thrive as you get older, you can move on to Chapter 4, where you will learn how you can take care of your brain as you get older.

4

NEUROPLASTICITY

As you get older, taking care of your brain is just as important as taking care of your physical health. According to Cynthiam (2021), your genetics only influence 25% of the way you age, while the remaining 75% is determined by your environment, behavior, and lifestyle—factors that you have control, or at least influence over. A study was conducted on a group of random individuals (aged between 57 and 71-years-old) and found that after using strategic brain exercises, these individuals experienced improved brain function after only 12 hours, with an additional 8% improvement in their blood flow and other measurements related to brain function (Wilson, 2014).

This research demonstrates that it **is** possible for a person to improve their brain's neuroplasticity at *any* age. It's quite simple to achieve, too. Improving brain function means keeping your brain constantly engaged as you get older. Learn new skills, take up a new hobby, exercise, and get involved with other people. This doesn't mean that you can't take a day off to relax or enjoy time to yourself, it simply means that it's important that you take part in activities that allow your brain to work and captivate your attention—whether you have retired or not. But what exactly is *neuroplasticity* and *why* is it so important?

WHAT IS NEUROPLASTICITY?

The brain has the ability to create the neurons needed to grow new neural networks when you enter a situation and learn new things. Connections between these networks can be adapted, allowing your neural pathways to re-organize and create new connections that give you the ability to learn and grow from these experiences. This helps you improve your ability to think, respond to a situation faster and more appropriately, and even listen better. Commonly known as *neuroplasticity,* these are only some of the benefits that are created as a result of your brain's ability to change and adapt as you get older and experience life. Neuroplasticity is made up of two main types of plasticity.

- **Structural plasticity:** When you are in a situation that allows you to gain new experiences and learn, your brain is able to change its structure to adapt to and remember these experiences. This allows you to use what you learned in similar situations, as well as be able to apply this new knowledge and skills to help you thrive in future situations. The more that you reflect on the memory—or practice the new skill—the stronger these new connections will become, allowing you to grow.
- **Functional plasticity:** As careful as you are, the unexpected does happen. If your brain is injured, or you experience some type of brain trauma like a stroke, the functions that are normally performed by the damaged area of your brain can be moved to an undamaged area. This type of plasticity plays an important role in helping you recover from head injuries—although, there are limits. For example, if one of your senses—like your sight—is damaged or lost, your other senses will become enhanced to help you cope with this loss and ensure your continued survival.

Neuroplasticity is extremely important for your brain's continued functioning as well as your survival in a world that is constantly changing and requires you to adapt and change with it. You may be getting older, but that doesn't mean you will stop learning. It just looks different from the learning you are familiar with. Take part in your life and actively engage your brain, especially with things that interest you. As such, you need to understand how this ability works so that you can use it effectively, in a way that is suitable to both your interests and lifestyle.

How Does It Work?

During your first few years of life, your brain undergoes rapid growth. As you go from being a newborn who can't support their own head, to a toddler that is learning how to run around and climb on everything you really shouldn't be climbing on, it makes sense. Cherry (2022) explains that when you are born, the neurons found in your brain's cerebral cortex (the part of your brain responsible for learning, language, motor function, processing of sensory information, intelligence, and personality) are estimated to contain about 2,500 synapses (the area found between your neurons that allows for the relaying of nerve impulses). By the time you reach three-years-old, your synapses should have grown to about 15,000 per neuron (Cherry, 2022).

However, most adults have nearly half this number of synapses. Why? Well, when you go through life and experience new things, some of these connections are strengthened the more you use them, while others die because they aren't being used. As concerning as this may seem, it is normal and is referred to as *synaptic pruning.* The principles surrounding this can be explained using the example of learning a new skill like playing the guitar. The more you practice playing the guitar, the better you will sound and the easier it will be to play, but if you don't practice this new skill or practice rarely, you will see little to no improvements—perhaps losing this skill altogether. The development of new connections, and the pruning of weak ones allow your brain to adapt appropriately to your environment and lifestyle, helping you grow and thrive in a way that is both appropriate and unique to you. As such, neuroplasticity has many benefits.

Benefits of Neuroplasticity

The benefits of neuroplasticity explained in this section are quite broad, and the list is not necessarily complete, as everyone is affected by neuroplasticity differently. You may even experience benefits that aren't listed here. The overall aim of this section is to show you that taking care of your brain and its health will benefit you more than ignoring it and hoping for the best. It really is worth the effort that you put in. The list that follows will briefly explain the more common benefits of neuroplasticity that you may experience (Cherry, 2022).

- It provides your brain with the ability to change and adapt as you move through life and experience new things, allowing you to learn and grow.
- Allows your brain to revive or restore certain functions that may have been neglected, including skills like playing an instrument, dancing, or knitting.
- You are able to heal and recover—to a certain degree—from traumatic brain injuries.
- The improvement of your ability to remember, reason, and think. These three abilities are also known as your cognitive capabilities.
- It also allows certain areas of your brain to regain their strength and ability to function that they lost—either due to lack of use or injury.

Characteristics of Neuroplasticity

The benefits of neuroplasticity can be used to help you maintain the health of your brain and keep your mind sharp as you get older. Additionally, it has three key characteristics that play an important role in understanding how neuroplasticity works and how you can use it to improve your own brain's growth. These three key characteristics are explained below.

Your Brain's Capacity for Plasticity Is Limited

The degree to which you can shape and influence your brain is, unfortunately, limited. Certain areas of your brain play an important role in specific activities that ensure your body is functioning properly, including areas that have a critical role in speech, language, cognition, and movement. If an important area in the brain is damaged, a loss will occur that cannot be completely taken over by another part of your brain. Remember, if you lose your eyesight, no other part of your body can see; however, your other senses will often become enhanced to try and make up for your lack of sight and ensure your continued survival.

Environment and Age Play a Role

From the moment you are born, your brain undergoes a great number of changes. While your brain's ability for plasticity is present throughout your life, certain changes do have a more dominant role at certain life stages. When you go through puberty, for example, your hormones can influence your behavior, mood, and how your body functions. This helps your immature brain transition from childhood to adolescence, and through to adulthood (although a number of additional stages occur throughout these main stages of life). It allows you to constantly grow, change, and mature in a way that helps you adapt to your new age and stage in life. Additionally, your environment and genetics can also influence your brain's neuroplasticity to a certain degree.

Neuroplasticity Is Ongoing

The brain's ability to change, grow, and adapt through neuroplasticity involves many different types of cells. As such, it's an ongoing process. Your ability to learn means that your brain never stops changing in both structure and function. Additionally, when certain areas of the brain are injured, for whatever reason, the healthier parts of your brain will start to take over their functions—to a certain degree—restoring or changing your abilities and senses in a way that allows you to continue living your life.

NEUROPLASTICITY AS YOU AGE

New pathways and neural connections are formed in your brain when you learn and experience new things, ensuring that your brain's default mode of operation is constantly changing and improving. You need a *growth mindset* in order to effectively utilize your brain's capacity for neuroplasticity. This mindset involves actively believing that you have the ability to get better, smarter, and more skilled at an activity or skill through sustained effort, despite your age and current abilities. However, neuroplasticity does change as you get older. Neuroplasticity is often less observed in adults because, unlike children, we aren't constantly working to actively improve and hone this ability. As you work through this guide, remember that your brain does have the capacity for great change; however, **you** need to be willing to continuously sustain the effort it takes to improve your neuroplasticity and do your best to live a healthy life.

Improve Your Brain's Neuroplasticity

As fragile as it can be, the brain is actually quite resilient, partly due to its capacity for neuroplasticity. As research is still being conducted on this ability, a number of tools and techniques have been developed to promote neuroplasticity and brain health as you get older. These strategies can be used by anyone, at any age, to help you exercise your brain and maintain your cognitive functioning as you get older. The brain's continued ability to change as you move through life affects everyone differently, especially because your brain is constantly reorganizing its pathways and connections in response to your unique life experiences. You can enhance your cognitive abilities, improve your ability to learn, and strengthen the areas of your brain where age-related cognitive decline commonly occurs. Getting older doesn't mean you become powerless. Armed with the knowledge and tools in this guide, you *can* train your brain and help it adapt and change as you experience new things. However, before you move on to the steps that will help you improve your brain plasticity, you need to remember two important tips:

- **Get enough sleep:** Throughout the process of improving your neuroplasticity, you need to ensure that you are getting enough sleep so that your brain can rest and recuperate. This is important for both your physical and cognitive health. You should be getting at least seven and a half hours of sleep every night.
- **Exercise your brain:** Essentially, the activities that you use to help improve your cognition should capture your attention and help you focus it, allowing you to actively stimulate changes in your brain. How certain activities impact you will change as you get older. Once you notice that you are no longer as interested

in the activity, simply adjust to your brain's new needs. Exercising your brain could involve activities such as learning a new language or instrument, exploring new places, dancing, reading, knitting, or drawing, for example.

If your family has a history of age-related diseases—specifically neurodegenerative diseases—it's important that you introduce the steps to improving your brain's plasticity as early as possible. While they cannot prevent neurodegenerative diseases, they are helpful in strengthening your brain and improving its health so that the symptoms or effects of these diseases may be lessened; however, the results differ among individuals and cannot be guaranteed (Smith, 2013).

Steps to Better Brain Plasticity

Before moving onto the steps for improving your brain's neuroplasticity, you need to understand that your brain is split into two hemispheres: The right and left hemisphere. Each side of your brain is responsible for certain activities, as well as controlling a specific side of your body. The left hemisphere controls the right side of your body and is responsible for controlling logical thought processes, including the ability to perceive objects, analyze your thoughts, and any other logical process that your brain carries out.

The right hemisphere of your brain controls the left side of your body and is responsible for interpreting your emotions and nonverbal expressions. Additionally, it helps you to recognize the overall pattern of something—like during reading activities. It's important that the exercises and activities that you use to improve your brain's neuroplasticity utilize both sides of your brain simultaneously as often as possible. Examples involve ambidextrous activities like knitting, playing a musical instrument, or sculpting with clay. Using the knowledge that you have gained in this chapter, follow the nine steps below to help you improve your brain's neuroplasticity.

Step One: Use Your Entire Brain and Engage in Challenges

The best way to engage in new challenges consistently is to set goals for yourself that you can pursue as you get older. These goals don't have to be big or life changing; they can be as simple as learning a new skill and then using that skill to create something meaningful for yourself. Learning the skills needed to bind books and then binding a journal that you made for a friend is an example of how you can set up your goals in a way that continuously challenges you and keeps you engaged while allowing you to do something that is meaningful and interesting.

First, you need to gain clarity. Essentially, determining what it is that you want to do as you get older will help you set meaningful goals that you can stick to. In the case of this guide, your goals may include learning about anti-aging techniques and how to implement them successfully, and then using these techniques to improve your health and well-being. You have to be willing to consistently engage in new challenges, learn, and actively take part in activities. If you aren't willing to put in the work, you won't experience any of neuroplasticity's benefits. Working on activities that help you partake and feel fulfilled will increase your chances of continuing these behaviors, challenging your brain, and improving your neuroplasticity successfully as you get older.

Step Two: Practice Focused Attention

It's important that the goals and activities that you work on capture your attention. If you aren't interested in something but you're doing it because it's supposed to help you, it's pointless. Your attention will start to wander, and your brain won't be focused on or engaged with the task. As such, you won't experience any improvements in your neuroplasticity. You can also practice focused attention when you have conversations, experience new things, or go about your daily life. Reflect on what these situations taught you or even what you heard. This practice has many benefits and helps you actively increase the connections between both sides of your brain.

After gaining clarity in the step above, reflect on your passions, hobbies, and other interests that you had to put aside when you were younger in order to attend to your responsibilities. Compile a list of these activities and rank them in order of the activities that interest you. It is helpful if these activities utilize both hemispheres of your brain simultaneously. After compiling this list, choose one activity and use it to help you start setting your goals. Goal setting is a tool that can help you engage in lifelong learning, which is critical for improving your neuroplasticity.

Step Three: Approach Each Activity as if You Are Experiencing It for the First Time

Don't try to achieve your entire goal in a short period of time. It will only overwhelm you and even put you off working toward your goal. Instead, break your goal down into smaller steps that allow you to work on it consistently every day. Smaller steps will also help you approach the activity as though you are experiencing everything for the first time. This can help you improve your neuroplasticity and nurture your mental health.

Allowing yourself to have a childlike wonder about the world, even if you are over the age of 50, can bring some of the magic back to your everyday life. This can make each day exciting and more enjoyable. Record your progress in a journal. Then reflect on your day or the activity you completed and try to find something good about it—this is similar to using a gratitude journal. Additionally, taking smaller steps that help you enjoy each day and activity will improve your confidence, help you feel accomplished, and motivate you to stay committed to your goal, ensuring lasting change.

Step Four: Exercise

Exercise is probably the one tip that is repeated in every bit of advice on improving your health and lifestyle, but there's a reason for that. It plays an important role in your mental and physical health by strengthening your body's circulation and reducing your stress levels, resulting in improved blood and oxygen flow to the brain and thereby aiding neuroplasticity. You should be exercising three to four days per week for thirty to forty-five minutes per session. There are several different types of exercises available. You can take part in a single type of exercise or combine and rotate them to ensure that you don't get bored. Weight training is a great way to work all your muscle groups. Cardio exercises help you improve your blood and oxygen flow and can capture your attention if you exercise outside or with friends. While balance exercises—like yoga or tai chi—are important as you get older and help decrease your risk of falling and hurting yourself accidentally.

Step Five: Protect Your Brain

There are a variety of activities that you can use to protect your brain. Mindfulness and meditation are the two most popular activities. Meditation has many benefits for your brain's structure, as it can increase the strength and thickness of the frontal cortex, which normally decreases with age, boost your immune system, and decrease your stress levels. Guided meditation videos and audios are available on CD and on sites like YouTube. You can also go to class or meditate at home.

Mindfulness is great for helping you increase your awareness of your surroundings and your own body and mind. This helps you notice your thought patterns, as well as what is happening in your body. It can help you improve your self-awareness and self-control to make meaningful decisions–strengthening your neuroplasticity. You can practice mindfulness using a gratitude journal, through yoga or tai chi, by focusing on your goals, and by sticking to a consistent morning routine.

Step Six: Develop Stimulating Friendships

Getting older doesn't mean you have to be lonely. Actively cultivating your current friendships and creating new, meaningful friendships is important for improving your neuroplasticity. It allows you to practice a range of skills, learn new things, stay engaged, and focus your attention. You have to remember that the more time you spend with someone, the more influence they will have on you, even if you don't notice it. Try to ensure that the people you are friends with have values that align with your own.

The people you spend time with should also encourage you to live your life, engage in meaningful experiences, focus on your health, and trigger the active decision-making part of your brain in a way that helps you grow for the better instead of holding you back or hurting you. A great way to make new friends is to join group activities or clubs that focus on things that interest you, like a bird watchers' group, knitting club, book club, sports club, or even a group that walks or hikes together. You can also volunteer at your local library or anywhere you feel you will enjoy yourself.

Step Seven: Laugh Often

Laughing is all about embracing a positive attitude about life, which I discussed in detail in chapter two.

Having a positive mindset can help you reduce your stress levels and naturally improve your well-being. If you are joking around with friends and family using humor that mentally challenges you, it can help you improve your neuroplasticity as it keeps you engaged and alert.

Step Eight: Stop Procrastinating

Whether you are working on your goals, improving your neuroplasticity using other activities, or generally implementing the anti-aging strategies in this guide, you need to become aware of when you are procrastinating and work to actively stop. Procrastinating prevents you from living your life, but it often has an underlying source, such as fear of failure or other insecurities. You have to make conscious decisions on purpose when you notice that you are procrastinating.

When you get an idea or want to work on an activity, start counting backwards from five. As you count, take steps to implement the idea or activity in some way—whether that's setting up for taking action, writing down the idea, or putting on your walking shoes—ensure that whatever you do will help you take the next step to working on the activity. Essentially, you need to pre-plan your activity and take action, then you can make a decision before allowing yourself to acknowledge your feelings about whether you want to do it or not. This will also help you stop your brain from killing ideas as soon as they arise and decrease the number of times you procrastinate instead of doing what you want to do.

Step Nine: Raise Your Standards

You need to have higher standards for yourself, but they also need to be realistic; otherwise, you will actively set yourself up for failure. Reflect on your abilities and goals. Decide which goals you want to pursue and set yourself up to achieve them. Proactively take preventative measures against your procrastination and ignore what others say. Getting older doesn't mean you are less capable of doing something. Take care of yourself now so that your future self can reap the benefits. This includes holding yourself accountable and being consistent.

You may not be perfect or immediately succeed, but the fact that you tried and did your best is more important than not even trying in the first place. By actively engaging in your life and working on improving and maintaining the health of your brain, you will be well on your way to taking advantage of your brain's capacity for plasticity.

KEY TAKEAWAYS

- As you get older, it's important that you take care of your brain's health.
- By utilizing your brain's capacity for plasticity, you can keep your brain engaged and maintain its health.
- You can improve your neuroplasticity at any age.
- By understanding how neuroplasticity works, its benefits, and characteristics, you can effectively use it to improve your overall health and well-being.
- There are nine basic steps that you can use to effectively improve your brain's capacity for plasticity in a way that suits your interests, goals, and lifestyle.

While the brain can be difficult to understand, knowing how to improve its health is an important step in the anti-aging process. It helps you introduce a number of strategies that are beneficial for your overall health. These methods also have additional benefits, like decreasing your stress levels. In chapter five, you will learn how stress can fast-forward the aging process and what you can do to combat it.

5

STRESS FAST-FORWARDS AGING

How you age is affected by how you experience stress. In general, stress negatively impacts the aging process. You are probably tired of being told that you need to learn to relax and take time for yourself because "stress is bad." As often as you hear this phrase —and as annoying as it can become—it's also true. Stress impacts a variety of factors in your life, including your mental and physical health. In terms of the aging process, it can affect *how* you age as well as the *speed* at which you age, on both a cellular and surface level. So, what exactly is *stress*?

A variety of definitions for stress exist, and the one used is often based on how stress applies to that situation. However, a general definition of stress explains how this natural mental and physical response occurs when you are exposed to an outside stimulus—also known as a *stressor*—that impacts your body's normal balance. While this is known as the *stress response,* you may also hear it called the *fight or flight* response. Essentially, when you are exposed to a stressor that poses a threat to your mental or physical safety—possibly both—your body will trigger this mechanism to ensure that you will survive the situation with little to no harm. This stress response doesn't go away or become less active as you get older because its main aim is to ensure your continued survival, allowing you to adapt as your surroundings change, but its effect on your body will change as you get older.

When your stress response is activated, your body will react and manifest symptoms in a manner that is different from the response of another person; however, there are a few common symptoms or reactions that occur among many people, regardless of their age. Your heart rate will increase to ensure that your blood moves faster throughout your body to ensure you are getting enough oxygen, increasing your blood pressure, and breathing, as well as helping your muscles prepare to react as fast as possible. In a situation where your stress takes the form of a deadline or having a busy day, you may find that you can't sleep, that your digestive system is upset and slower than normal, or that you might become sick due to a suppressed immune system. These are all normal reactions to stress, and in a dangerous situation, they can be beneficial as they help you cope and survive.

Unfortunately, when being stressed out becomes your natural state of being—also called *chronic stress*—your mind and body may be impacted more severely. Your body will find it difficult to regulate itself, causing it to break down on a cellular level, making it difficult for your organs to function properly and triggering health issues like headaches, diabetes, heart disease, asthma, gastrointestinal issues, or even triggering mental health issues like depression and anxiety. To properly understand the effect of stress on aging and how you can effectively manage it, you first need to understand how it affects your mind and body as a whole.

STRESS AND THE BIOLOGICAL CLOCK

Stress is a natural part of life, and you are exposed to it every day. Your biological clock, however, can be affected by the type of stress you are exposed to. In simple terms, the biological clock is your body's mechanism that controls the timing of body processes and physiological states, such as aging. Your body has natural defense mechanisms against stress that it uses to help you cope and survive. As you get older, these mechanisms start to break down. Unfortunately, that means that the negative impact that stress has on your mental and physical well-being increases.

Physical stress can manifest in situations where you find it difficult to adjust to temperature changes—like being more sensitive to the cold or the heat—or you may find it more difficult to recover from physical exercise, especially when you previously had no issues. This doesn't mean that you need to avoid such situations. You simply need to cater to your body's new needs and learn how to manage these physical stressors in a healthy way. Mental or emotional stress is often more subtle and difficult to identify until its impact on your health and well-being is already serious. The consequences of both types of stress—especially when it's chronic—can be quite severe, but that doesn't mean that you are helpless. So, what is the connection between stress and the aging process?

Connection Between Stress and Aging

In a study conducted on a New Haven community of 444 individuals, aged between 18 and 50, it was found that large amounts of stress can be linked to faster rates of aging (Jagoo, 2022). There are a variety of reasons for this, but two of the main factors studied included emotional regulation and behavioral factors, like smoking and weight. Unfortunately, more research needs to be conducted on this topic to provide us with a more detailed understanding of the effects of stress on the aging process, but we do know that stress can impact how you age (Jagoo, 2022).

How Stress Affects the Body

When you are exposed to stress, an alarm is set-off in your body that signals the release of stress hormones—like cortisol and adrenaline—into your body so that you can react appropriately. The levels of such hormones are generally quite high in such situations, and when the alarm turns off (once the stressor has been dealt with), these levels are supposed to return to normal so that your body can return to its balanced state. If the stress you experience or are exposed to is chronic, however, your system is thrown off-balance due to an overload of stress-hormones in your body. When such hormones are present for long periods, they can trigger health issues, or exacerbate current illnesses, such as weakening your immune system, increasing your blood pressure, or contributing to heart disease. Additionally, this new state of being impacts your brain, and it becomes difficult for your hormone levels to be properly regulated.

This can be especially dangerous as you get older. Your stress response slowly breaks down, and large amounts of stress will become more harmful the older you get, causing them to have a greater impact on your health. For example, when cortisol—a steroid hormone that plays a role in your metabolism and the functioning of your immune system—is produced in large amounts for long periods of time, your hippocampus becomes negatively impacted. The hippocampus is the part of your brain responsible for the storage and retrieval of your memories. When it's negatively impacted, you may find that you struggle to remember or recall things, resulting in memory-related issues and possibly increasing your risk of Alzheimer's disease.

After years of being constantly exposed to stress and having high levels of stress hormones, the rate at which you age will start to increase, causing your immune cells to become damaged, but you can do something about it. You need to learn how to manage your stress in a healthy way so that you can reduce its impact on your mind and body.

Impact of Mood Regulation on Stress

The New Haven study demonstrated that your ability to regulate your emotions and control yourself can also impact how stress affects the aging process and your well-being (Jagoo, 2022). Individuals with mood and anxiety disorders will often engage in certain activities to help them cope with stress. In reality, these activities were found to contribute to their stress levels. When these individuals went to therapy and began taking medications to help them, they felt happier and able to participate in, and give back to, their community (Jagoo, 2022).

As such, therapy and medication may be able to help individuals with poor emotional regulation cope more effectively with stress. When you are able to improve how you manage stress, you improve your mental capabilities, your relationships, and your ability to respond in a healthier manner when faced with a stressful situation. Additional benefits of effective stress management include eating well and exercising—which contribute to a healthier lifestyle and improve the aging process—as well as lowering your cholesterol levels and blood pressure which can improve your longevity and may boost your immune system's functioning, thus decreasing the frequency and severity of illnesses.

Stress Isn't Always Bad

Did you know that stress can be split up into two types: Good and bad stress? It may be surprising, but not all stress is bad for you. Good stress helps you stay motivated when working towards a goal, improves your performance, and can inspire you. Examples of good stress include the approaching deadline on a project for work, being nervous before a presentation or speech, or taking part in fun challenges with friends. Good stress can help you grow, but it can become bad stress that negatively impacts your health if you continuously experience it.

Chronic stress can result in bad stress—the type of stress many of us are familiar with. Bad stress impacts you both mentally and physically. It often results from situations where you don't have any control, or you become distressed, including being let go, losing someone you care about, or remembering bad memories. Stress has the ability to increase the rate at which you age, especially as you get older. This can impact your quality of life and health.

Essentially, stress has the power to shape your life, but **you** have the ability to determine if you will accommodate such stress or remove it. First, you need to work on identifying the sources of stress in your life—both good and bad—before deciding how you will manage it. There are a multitude of management techniques available, including exercise. Stress may have the ability to speed up the aging process, but improving your emotional regulation, self-control, and stress management techniques can help you reduce its impact on your well-being.

STRESS ACCELERATES AGING

Stress doesn't only impact your body on a physical level, it also has the ability to affect you on a cellular level. Your ability to respond to stress is an adaptive mechanism that often operates at the nervous system level. This mechanism helps your body return to its balanced state after the temporary threat has been dealt with. Often associated with inflammation in the body due to psychological stress, oxidative stress is one of the main factors that have a destructive effect on your body. It's also one of the reasons why chronic stress can accelerate the aging process (Yegerov et al., 2020).

An overproduction of reactive oxygen species (ROS) can result in oxidative stress. ROS can damage various tissues in your body and are mainly found in your mitochondria; however, they are normally suppressed by mitochondrial mutations. When macrophages (tissue cells with the ability to destroy bacteria and viruses, and form part of the immune system) are introduced into the situation, they can cause inflammation that is specific to the aging process known as *inflammaging*.

Inflammaging is a state of being where your body experiences chronic inflammation, often resulting from stress. This type of inflammation is associated with the aging process and results in chronic, asymptomatic, low-grade inflammation that contributes to a number of age-related diseases such as hypertension, atherosclerosis, and diabetes (Yegorov et al., 2020). When macrophages encourage inflammation, they aim to trigger the immunity you had to certain bacteria and viruses before you were even born so that you can combat that stressor. When you experience chronic stress, your cells are unable to regulate this process properly and return to their normal state, resulting in chronic inflammation that can further increase the rate at which you age.

Aging Due to Psychological Stress

Psychological stress further increases your risk of developing a variety of diseases, both related and unrelated to the aging process. Oxidative stress has been linked to accelerated aging and psychological stress that results from mental health issues like post-traumatic stress disorder (PTSD) and major depressive disorder (Yegerov et al., 2020). This is partly due to the role that cellular senescence plays as a result of inflammation triggered by oxidative stress, and it can increase your risk of cancer, neurodegenerative and autoimmune disorders, and cardiovascular disease (Yegerov et al., 2020).

Impact of Cellular Senescence and Cellular Aging

Cellular senescence can be triggered by chronic stress, making it difficult for your body to return to its regular state of being. Additionally, the occurrence of oxidative stress increases the loss of telomeric DNA, impacting your body in a manner that is similar to the effects of regular cellular senescence.

Understanding how stress affects your whole body helps explain *why* it increases the rate at which you age, as well as *how* you age. While it's annoying to constantly hear friends, family members, and even healthcare professionals tell you to reduce your stress levels, their advice is valid. But it's not always as simple as decreasing the amount of stress you experience, especially in a world that is changing every day. Instead, you need to learn how to effectively manage your stress in a way that works for you.

STRESS MANAGEMENT

Managing your stress levels doesn't need to involve any extravagant activities or going out of your way to do something. These management tools actually involve a lot of the wellness tips mentioned in previous chapters as well as the strategies that will be mentioned in future chapters. As such, I would recommend that after going through this guide, you note down all the activities that you are interested in and identify any overlaps that could cover more than one aspect of anti-aging, like exercising and mindfulness meditation. You could even create your own activities that cover more than one aspect but are more suitable to your lifestyle. The information provided in this book is meant to act as your *guide* to anti-aging and not as a strict rule book. Remember that we all lead different lives, and what works for one person won't work for another. Do what is best for you and your well-being. The strategies that I discussed below are the most common and effective methods that are used for managing stress.

Strategies for Managing Stress

Using the strategies below, create a stress management plan that you can use to help you cope with and manage your stress levels. Having a set plan can make it easier to use the activities to help you. You can even change this plan as you identify what methods work best for you. The strategies that follow are some of the more common stress management techniques that are practiced.

Style of Stress Management

How do you currently react to stress? You may find that you use a combination of healthy and unhealthy techniques for managing your stress, with varying effects. The aim of this tool is to help you identify how you currently deal with stress so that you can improve your well-being and decrease the impact of stress on your mind and body. The methods below are healthy management tools. You can use them to help you create a management style that suits your lifestyle and goals. You can write the methods that you would like to use in a step-by-step action plan, or you can create a list of techniques, and hang it up in an area of your home that you frequently walk past. Remember that the types of strategies that you use should be appropriate for your lifestyle. As such, whether you are currently retired, still working, or run your own business, you need to consider how this will affect your stress levels and how you can manage them appropriately.

Exercise

Chapter four explained how you can introduce exercise into your lifestyle to improve your neuroplasticity. It's applicable here too. Exercise is a great way to physically get rid of stress at any age. It also has many benefits, including helping you remain independent and strong as you get older, managing your cortisol levels so that its effects are reduced, encouraging the regeneration of new brain cells, improving your brain health, and increasing your bone density, lung capacity, and longevity.

Body Manipulation

Physically moving your body is important for your overall health and well-being, but body manipulation also has several benefits. While its movements are more subtle, this type of exercise can have a big impact on reducing your stress levels. It physically affects your body by reducing the physical impact of stress, reducing your blood pressure, increasing your energy levels, improving brain function, and helping you maintain your sense of independence. Examples of body manipulation include:

- **Massage:** When a qualified individual manipulates your muscles and tissues through physical actions such as rubbing, kneading, or tapping for therapeutic or relaxation purposes (Merriam-Webster, n.d.-i).
- **Yoga:** Special breathing techniques and physical postures that are performed with the aim of improving your well-being—both mentally and physically (Merriam-Webster, n.d.-n).

- **Tai Chi:** A system of special exercises consisting of meditative movements (Merriam-Webster, n.d.-m).
- **Reiki:** A qualified and experienced practitioner will use their hands to touch and manipulate your body's natural energy fields to improve your overall well-being (Merriam-Webster, n.d.-l).
- **Craniosacral therapy:** A type of touch therapy that aims to improve the functioning of the bones, tissues, fluids, and membranes that surround—or are associated with—the brain and spinal cord (Merriam-Webster, n.d.-b).

Mindfulness

As discussed in Chapter 4, this method is a primary stress management technique. Through activities like meditation, mindfulness helps you decrease your stress levels, improve your brain function, and become more aware of both your body and surroundings. Additionally, it helps you take notice of your thoughts and attitude in a specific situation, helping you shift to a more positive outlook.

Eating Right

Diet plays an important role in your overall health, but it's also important for managing your stress levels.

When foods lack nutritional density (like fast foods), your body struggles to extract the vitamins, minerals, energy, and other nutritional factors that allow your body to function optimally. As such, speak with a dietician and your healthcare provider to assess how your current diet is benefiting you and what you can do to improve it. This may include introducing supplements, as discussed in Chapter 3, to make up for any nutritional needs that you cannot meet. Remember, we all have different diets, and the food available to you will differ year-round.

Generally, a nutritional diet is low in carbohydrates, contains saturated fats that benefit your health, and contains large amounts of eggs, poultry, nuts, vegetables, meat, and fish. Additionally, try to avoid excessive amounts of sugar in your diet. It would be best to discuss with a dietician how much sugar is safe for you, depending on the sugar levels found in the foods that you are currently eating, like fruits and carbohydrates. Everyone has different needs for sugar, especially if they have health problems like diabetes, so I wouldn't recommend giving up sugar completely before talking to a doctor about it.

Pre-Plan Activities

Whether you have already retired or not, you need to plan activities that provide you with stimulation and a sense of fulfillment. These factors are important for your mental health and can help you manage your stress levels. In a working environment, you are provided with this type of stimulation daily, but when you retire, you may feel lost without it. Engage in social activities that take place weekly, like book clubs, cooking classes, volunteering at a museum, or even going back to school to learn a new skill.

Carry On Working

If you are not a fan of sitting still or being idle, then think about doing part-time work, becoming a consultant for a company, volunteering, or even starting your own business. While it's best to lay the groundwork for such activities at least five years before retiring, you could still pursue such opportunities if you have already retired. Retiring doesn't mean you can no longer do anything or be part of society. It simply means that you now have more control over how you will be spending your time.

Cultivate Your Community

As discussed in detail in chapters four and seven, developing your social circle can be helpful in giving you the support you need when you feel stressed. As such, being a part of a supportive community that allows you to actively participate can keep you mentally sharp, decrease your risk of memory related issues, lower the amount of stress hormones in your body, and even improve your longevity.

Stay Present in Reality

It doesn't matter if the thing that is stressing you out is real, imaginary, or a future or anticipated problem because your brain is unable to tell the difference. This means that you will experience the same amount of stress with the same negative impact regardless of when this stressor occurs. Use your stress management plan and activities like mindfulness meditation to help you stay in the present moment. Having a set plan can give you a sense of control over a situation, reducing the impact of stress on your mind and body.

Many of the methods mentioned above have been explained in detail in previous chapters. This demonstrates that you don't have to perform a vast number of different steps every day to experience the anti-aging benefits you have been pursuing. You simply need to identify the common activities, combine them with the strategies that don't appear more than once, and then create your own anti-aging plan that covers your overall health and well-being. Essentially, the key to anti-aging is taking care of yourself and enjoying your life, regardless of your age.

KEY TAKEAWAYS

- Stress does have the ability to accelerate the aging process.
- You are affected mentally, physically, and on a cellular level by stress.
- Understanding how stress impacts your body will help you understand what you can do to effectively manage it and reduce its impact on your well-being.
- Not all stress is bad, but even too much good stress can be detrimental to your health.
- Use the stress management techniques to help you build a stress management plan that can be used when you are exposed to stressors.

Understanding how stress impacts your body and impacts the aging process can help you take better care of yourself as you get older. However, you shouldn't limit yourself to one location when taking care of yourself. Go outside and get in-touch with nature. Through activities like earthing, you can improve your mental and physical health, manage stress and anxiety, and address a variety of other health issues that both impact and result from the aging process. Chapter 6 will explain the anti-aging effects of earthing in more detail.

6

ANTI-AGING EFFECTS OF EARTHING

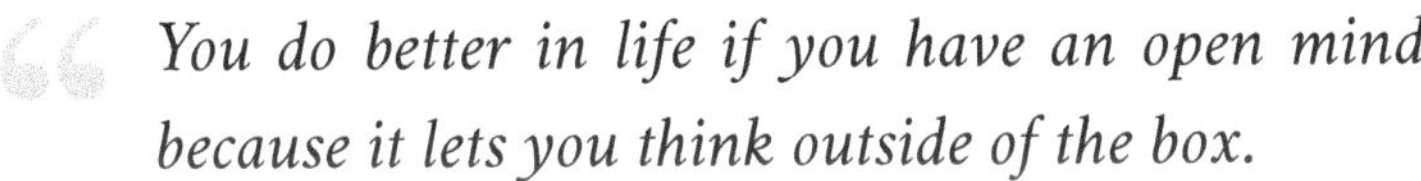

> *You do better in life if you have an open mind because it lets you think outside of the box.*
>
> — DAVID D MCCRAY

I understand if you feel skeptical about using the concept of getting in touch with nature as an anti-aging tool. In fact, it's normal for you to trust science and proven medical practices over what you probably feel is simply a new health trend. However, earthing has been studied in more detail over the years to understand if it's simply a new trend or if it has an actual, positive impact on your body. Studying the history of earthing shows that this health practice isn't new. It's actually an ancient holistic practice that was used by our ancestors, long before we had the science and evidence, we have today to back it up (Ibe, 2022).

Additionally, earthing is still a topic of interest in the scientific community, and new information is constantly becoming available. You have to remember that, just like with normal medical treatments and medications, your experience with earthing will differ compared to others. All you have to do is allow yourself to approach this chapter with an open mind. This tool is essentially free (unless you decide to buy the earthing equipment discussed later in this chapter), so it won't cost you anything to learn about its history, how it works, as well as what the science says. Let's start by learning about what "earthing" is.

WHAT IS EARTHING?

"Earthing" is a concept often applied to anything involving wiring and electrical currents. Your home contains wiring that allows you to access electricity with the aim of switching on lights, using electrical devices like your oven, or using outlets to plug these devices in. The wiring found in households form a circuit that provides a path for electric currents to move through safely. However, this current may stray outside of its circuit, or a fault may occur that disrupts the circuit. In such situations, the electrical current needs somewhere to go. The circuit found in your home is connected to the earth which contains its own electrical currents—allowing the charge to be safely neutralized. This prevents electrical fires and other issues that could pose a threat to your home and your safety.

Grounding is actually a form of earthing that is practiced to directly connect the human body to the Earth's natural electric charge, with the purpose of stabilizing the electrical current found in the body. Essentially, you are applying similar principles to those used when wiring the home or other electrical devices to ensure their optimal and safe functioning. In this way, you are able to stabilize your body's electrical current so that it matches that of the Earth's current. This connection can take the form of bare skin contact with the Earth including the sand, soil, water, or grass. Earthing is a practice that often occurs when a person intends to improve their mental well-being and reduce their stress levels and pain. While it may seem like this is a new practice, it actually has roots in ancient indigenous societies.

History of Earthing

Its name may have differed across the globe, but earthing was practiced by our ancestors—both on purpose and unknowingly—as a result of the lifestyles they led. The clothes they wore, often consisting of animal skins and natural fibers, allowed them to stay in constant contact with the Earth. Our ancestors also chose to remove their shoes and walk around barefoot when they could. The contact between their bare skin and the Earth allowed for an exchange of electrons—these electrons have been found to have anti-inflammatory and other anti-aging properties—that helped them stabilize their body's natural rhythms with the Earth's (Holford, 2022; Ibe, 2022). This direct contact with the Earth allowed them to take advantage of its natural healing powers and improve their health and well-being. They may not have had the science we do today to back it up, but our ancestors were observant and smart enough to figure out that this behavior could impact their body's state of being.

In 1891, earthing was considered part of a "newer healing science" and was studied by Louis Kuhne before science began to advise and encourage people to take time every day to go outside and connect with the Earth on purpose (Ibe, 2022).

An American medical doctor, George Starr White, was one of the scientists to start investigating how earthing could impact things like the quality of sleep. His experiment involved grounding his test subjects by using copper wires (that have the ability to conduct electricity) attached to his test subjects and the pipes found in their home. His findings suggested that earthing could have a positive impact on a person's quality of sleep (Ibe, 2022).

Research is still being conducted on earthing, how it works, and its effects. As technology advances and scientists are able to gather more detailed information, they have been able to better investigate the effects of grounding on the human body. Overall, it's been found that the electrons that naturally occur in the Earth have the ability to balance the electrical current found in the human body (Ibe, 2022). This can be beneficial for your health and the aging process, but I will expand more on this later in the chapter. First, let's take a look at the different types of earthing available.

Types of Earthing

In the present, we are often cut-off from the Earth's electrical field more often than not as a result of our lifestyle choices, such as wearing insulated shoes, living in multi-story buildings, and lacking access to natural environments and surfaces—like grass, soil, and lakes. Additionally, your life is vastly different from that of your ancestors. That doesn't mean that you won't be able to practice this anti-aging technique. It may actually be one of the easier tools to use. The different types of earthing available all have one thing in common: Direct contact between your skin and the Earth itself. While you can choose the type of grounding strategies that suit your lifestyle, the list below includes a variety of ways that you can practice earthing every day.

- Swim in a lake or the ocean.
- Walk on the grass or sand barefoot.
- Stand in the wet sand surrounding bodies of water like lakes and the ocean.
- Lay on your back in your garden or at the park.
- Work in your garden and get your hands dirty by digging around in the soil.

- Take a bath.
- Use grounding equipment like grounding mats, blankets, or patches and socks.

Please note: Regardless of the type of earthing being practiced, please take the necessary precautions to ensure your safety, especially when going swimming or walking around barefoot.

Importance of Earthing

At first glance, earthing may appear to be a straightforward topic, but the history and science behind this ancient practice can become quite complicated. Don't worry, you don't need to try and decipher special scientific terms in order to understand the importance of this practice. You already know that the aging process is affected by the presence of inflammation in your body and its severity from previous chapters. Remember that inflammation often stems from the oxidative processes that occur throughout your body; as such, the health and functioning of your body's normal processes—also known as *physiological processes* —can be impacted.

An accumulation of positive ions—atoms with the ability to carry a charge—either positive or negative (Merriam-Webster, n.d.-g)—often play a role in inflammatory processes. Antioxidants can be used to provide your body with the free electrons needed to neutralize the free radicals produced by oxidative stress; thereby, helping you restore balance to your body's systems. Earthing has the ability to directly provide your body with these electrons to successfully complete this process. So, how does earthing impact your body's regular functioning?

Effects of Earthing on Your Physiological Processes

Through an experiment used to determine what effect earthing has on the human body, scientists were able to determine that earthing has the ability to improve a number of your body's natural processes (Holford, 2022). Improvements were found in the body's electrolyte levels. Electrolytes are important for your body's optimal functioning, and these charged mineral particles are found in your bloodstream. Earthing prevented the clumping of red blood cells, contributing to improved heart health. Cortisol levels were also found to have been balanced, and melatonin levels improved. Melatonin is a powerful antioxidant that plays an important role in sleep and sleeps quality. Additionally, this experiment found a decrease in the presence of inflammation in the body (Holford, 2022).

The experiment supported the idea that your cell's electrical potential can be influenced by earthing (Holford,

2022). This influence prevents your blood cells from clumping together, allowing them to be "free flowing." Such cells are associated with improved blood and oxygen circulation, improved blood pressure, and a decreased risk of blood clots. Its impact also extends to pain reduction by decreasing inflammation, muscle stiffness, and improving your quality of sleep. As such, studies conducted on earthing have found that this practice can positively impact your body's physiological processes (Holford, 2022).

Impact of Earthing on the Effect of Electromagnetic Fields on the Body

Earthing has the ability to manipulate and change the electrical charges and current in the human body. Your continuous exposure to the electromagnetic fields created by everyday devices like cell phones, televisions, transformers, and Wi-Fi can influence your body's energy field and electrical charge, damaging your cells and tissues without you even knowing. Earthing has the ability to repair this damage to some degree (Halford, 2022).

Benefits of Earthing

Earthing has a variety of benefits, but it does take quite a bit of practice before you will start to experience these benefits. The list below provides you with a few of the main benefits of earthing.

- Reduction of inflammation in your body.
- Improved circulation.
- Lower levels of pain that were caused by chronic inflammation.
- Improved immune function.
- Hormonal and metabolic processes regain their balance.
- Improved quality of sleep.
- Positive impact on individuals who have cardiovascular disease.
- Improved mood and lower levels of depression and anxiety.
- Accelerated wound healing (Holford, 2020; Lockett, 2019; and Splichal, n.d.).

These are only some of the main benefits that earthing can provide you with. You may notice that these are also issues or conditions that are triggered by the aging process as discussed in previous chapters. As such, this practice does have a positive effect on the aging process. However, if you have any prior or current medical conditions, please be sure to seek the advice of your healthcare practitioner to ensure that there are no underlying causes before pursuing earthing as a healing practice.

How Can You Practice Earthing?

There are several ways that you can practice earthing. This tool is versatile and can be adapted to suit your lifestyle needs. The materials that are used today to build our lives often consist of insulated and non-conductive materials like rubber, vinyl, and plastic. Such materials cut you off from contact with the Earth. Eventually, this will start to impact your body negatively, especially the electrical current that is used to ensure your body's optimal functioning. You can use the resources available to you to practice earthing.

Earthing Using What Is Available to You

While it's important to take safety measures when working with conductive materials—as they allow for the flow of charged particles which can be dangerous—like copper, silver, and saltwater, these materials are typically used in a variety of earthing practices. A fine copper mesh is normally used in grounding mats and sheets, while beneficial sources of saltwater include saltwater lakes and the ocean. As such, you can choose the type of earthing practice that is suitable to your lifestyle and comfort levels.

You may even prefer to combine some of the different types of earthing practices. A great thing about this tool is that, unless you are buying earthing equipment, you don't actually have to spend money to experience its benefits.

Take 30 to 40 minutes every day to practice earthing. You could walk barefoot in your garden, on the beach, or at the park. Just be sure to check that the ground you are walking on doesn't have any broken glass or other hazardous objects. If you are feeling slightly more adventurous, try going swimming in a lake or the ocean if they are accessible to you. But try to visit places that have lifeguards and other safety precautions, and consider going with friends.

If you don't feel comfortable going for a swim, you can simply walk barefoot in the wet sand or soil surrounding the body of water. You will still be able to experience the same benefits of earthing that going for a swim would give you. Even gardening without gloves is a great way to practice this technique and increase your direct contact with the Earth. But what if you don't have the time, or access to, outdoor earthing resources?

Earthing Equipment

If you are unable to practice earthing outdoors—or don't have the time—you could invest in earthing equipment. These tools allow you to practice earthing indoors while you work or relax. Kindly note that the earthing equipment that you purchase will be set up, and work, differently depending on where you bought it from. I would suggest using sites like *YouTube* to help you investigate the various ways that earthing mats and sheets can be safely used and set up.

The conductive copper mesh found in this equipment is connected to the Earth through a grounding device. An Earthing rod is connected to your mat or sheet and then planted into the Earth (the soil in your garden), or plugged into the grounding mechanism on your wall socket.

In the United States (US), wall sockets have two straight slots where you would normally plug in an electrical device. This socket also has a third-round hole that functions as the grounding mechanism for your home's electrical circuit. The cord on your grounding mat or sheet should have a round plug that will only be able to fit into the round hole in the wall socket. You will be unable to plug a regular US, three-pronged plug into that socket at the same time. Simply put, the "plug" on your grounding mat or sheet will only fit into the ground of a regular U.S. prong outlet—this is the third hole found beneath where the two blades of a regular plug would fit (Amazon, 2022a).

You can either sleep the entire night with an earthing sheet, or use the mat for 30 to 40 minutes every day. It is ideal to combine these two methods if you cannot physically access a more natural environment often, but you should use the tool you are most comfortable with. Amazon sells earthing kits that you can use at home. These kits often come with detailed instructions and "how to" videos that will help you safely set up the equipment. However, you need to ensure that when you receive your kit, it has all the products listed online.

The website *grounded.com* has a variety of earthing equipment available for purchase, as well as a variety of options on how to connect your sheet or mat to the Earth. Additionally, they have detailed "how to" videos and tutorials on their site that will help you set up your kit easily and safely (Grounded, 2014).

ANTI-AGING EFFECTS OF EARTHING

It's important to understand how earthing can impact your overall well-being and improve your health, but you're probably wondering how any of this relates to anti-aging. Does earthing even have any anti-aging effects? Yes, it does! Acceleration of the aging process often results due to an increase in oxidative stress. Your exposure to free radicals only fuels this process further, increasing the presence of inflammation in your body. Instead of trying to cut out free radicals from your life —which is nearly impossible—you can manage and heal the damage they cause by providing them with the electrons they need through your contact with the Earth (Splichal, n.d.).

Frequent earthing can slow down the aging process and help you improve your overall well-being. Chronic inflammation typically occurs as you get older, accelerating the aging process and contributing to a number of age-related issues. As such, you need to decrease the impact of oxidative stress on your body. Remember that this type of stress is often caused by an imbalance of free radicals due to the accumulation of toxins in your body, which increases the severity of inflammation. Earthing can be used to combat this process, as it can neutralize the free radicals responsible for it (Splichal, n.d.). Let's look at the science behind earthing to better understand how it works and how it can impact the aging process.

What Does Science Say?

You currently have electricity flowing through your body, and you can use that to your advantage (Layton and Mancini, 2008). Earthing is a tool that can help you naturally restore and maintain your body's defense mechanisms as you get older; influencing your body's ability to heal, as well as the aging process (Lockett, 2019).

Through research and numerous experiments, scientists have been able to identify the positive impact of grounding equipment and earthing techniques on the human body. Additionally, the research conducted by Chevalier et al. (2012) supports the concept that Earth's free electrons can induce physiological changes in the human body that are beneficial to your health and well-being, including a positive effect on the aging process (Chevalier et al., 2012).

The environment in which you live impacts your health and how your body functions. Your lack of connection with the Earth can only further this impact, or you can use it to your advantage and improve your health by using the Earth's natural negative potential to regulate your body's own processes. The electrons found in antioxidants have the ability to neutralize free radicals. These electrons can be transferred from the Earth to your body through direct skin contact. Once absorbed, the electrons have the ability to neutralize the reactive oxygen species (ROS) involved in the oxidative process, allowing for a reduction in inflammation (Chevalier et al., 2012).

You are already aware that inflammation, especially if it's chronic, can impact how you age. Inflammation itself is impacted by the presence of ROS and your immune system, becoming a common symptom in age-related diseases and inflammaging. Earthing has anti-inflammatory effects that you can take advantage of. Through direct skin contact with the Earth, you will be able to absorb negatively charged antioxidant electrons into your body that have the ability to neutralize positively charged free radicals at the inflammation site (Chevalier et al., 2012).

In conclusion, the scientific studies that have been conducted on earthing and its effect on your well-being show that this tool *can* benefit your health. Additionally, it also has useful anti-aging effects that can help you manage and slow down the aging process. The best part is that this tool is easy to adapt to your lifestyle.

KEY TAKEAWAYS

- Earthing is an ancient healing practice.
- It involves direct skin contact with the Earth.
- The electrons that occur naturally in the Earth have the ability to help you balance your body's electrical currents.

- A variety of methods is available to practice earthing in a way that suits your lifestyle.
- Earthing can positively impact your body's normal processes, including the aging process.
- A number of benefits can be achieved by practicing earthing.
- If you can't access the outdoors easily—or it's unsafe—consider using grounding equipment to help you practice earthing indoors.

This practice may seem like some weird new fad, but its presence throughout history demonstrates how useful it was to our ancestors. If anything, it certainly won't hurt to go outside and walk around barefoot for a while. You may even make some new friends. Meaningful connections also play an important role in anti-aging, so move on to chapter seven and learn about their importance and how you can develop a meaningful connection with other people.

7

MEANINGFUL CONNECTIONS

As you get older, you may find that your social network—made up of friends, family, and acquaintances—becomes smaller. This is common as you start to realize that the relationships you want to keep in your life need to have meaning and positively impact your well-being. However, it's also common for aging to be framed by society as a lonely, isolated process. This false idea may make getting older seem even more unappealing than it actually is. But just because aging is made to look lonely, that doesn't mean it has to be. In fact, having meaningful connections with other people can play an important role in increasing your longevity and quality of life. Simply put, it's okay to care about other people, and it's important to let them care about you!

The appearance of the aging process being lonely often originates from the fact that as you get older, your social network normally becomes more tightly knit. Although, you may also find it harder to go out and meet new people, form new friendships, or reach out to old acquaintances. While it may be harder, that doesn't mean it's impossible. You are probably wondering why cultivating meaningful friendships is so important and how they could possibly have an impact on your lifespan.

IMPORTANCE OF MEANINGFUL CONNECTIONS

The strategies discussed throughout this guide takes a more direct approach to anti-aging. Basically, their focus is on your mental and physical health. When it comes to advise regarding anti-aging, many people will first tell you that you need to exercise, eat right, get enough sleep, and try to have a positive approach to life. While this advice isn't wrong, they are leaving out another key anti-aging technique: Taking the time to cultivate meaningful connections.

Meaningful connections simply involve your ability to connect with and relate to other people, including your friends, family, acquaintances, and even strangers that you come across in your daily life. Yes, it may sound strange, but you can have a meaningful and beneficial conversation when you compliment the earrings of the woman you met at the grocery store. That barely ten-second interaction counts as a meaningful connection. This doesn't mean that you have to go out and have conversations with everyone you meet. Firstly, that isn't safe, and secondly, if you aren't a very social person, it can be emotionally taxing.

Fortunately, even if your social network is small, you can still experience the same benefits that you would get by interacting with a variety of people. Even if you already have a close group of friends and family that you care about, you should still go out and allow yourself to interact with new people, make new connections, and cultivate friendships. Just do it on your own terms. As you get older, contact with other people starts to become more important, especially for your mental well-being. According to Senior Living (2020), not only are meaningful interactions important for your psychological and physical health, but they also have the ability to decrease your risk of cognitive decline, heart attacks, anxiety, and depression. They may even play a role in improving your lifespan. There are three key benefits to developing and maintaining meaningful relationships as you get older (Senior Living, 2020).

Sense of Worth

The friendships that you cultivate are the relationships that you choose to have in your life. As you get older, it may feel like you are losing control over a variety of things, including your ability to make your own decisions. This can create unwanted stress that impacts your self-control, self-esteem, and confidence. Fortunately, a meaningful relationship has the ability to counteract this negative impact. It also helps you feel more independent by improving how you see yourself as you get older. A large social network consisting of meaningful connections can improve your mental health and physical well-being. Additionally, the number of changes that occur as you get older can impact how you see yourself, but the friends and family members whose opinions you value can help you feel more confident about yourself despite these changes. Getting older doesn't mean you have to give in and stop living your life. How you live your life will just look different, and that's perfectly okay.

Exchange of Support

Having an established group of people that you can rely on will help you feel supported, especially when your life changes. In return, you will be able to support your friends regardless of whether they are older, younger, or even the same age as you. The people who form part of your social network can provide you with valuable support—especially when you need it the most—and an opportunity for social interaction that can combat feelings of loneliness and isolation as you get older. Additionally, it provides you with someone you can talk to, opportunities to get together and exchange stories and life experience over lunch, you can laugh with them, and you can even do things together—like go to the movies, take part in the same hobby you both enjoy, or even try out new hobbies together. This type of support takes away some of the fear that often accompanies the unknown, if you can do it with a friend.

Your central source of support may come from your family, spouse, and adult children. Unfortunately, we don't always move in the same direction as they do, especially as time passes by. This doesn't mean that they don't care about you. They simply have different interests. This gives you the opportunity to create your own new support network that helps you feel confident and supported, lowering your anxiety, and decreasing the occurrence of depression, while also increasing your self-esteem, sense of self-worth, and independence.

You will also be able to give back to your support network and provide them with the same care that they give you, but you can't do that unless you feel the same way about them. Being able to give back to the people that you care about will help you improve your well-being and give your life continued purpose. Compassion and concern for others can also protect against feelings of meaninglessness and loneliness. Brief connections to relative strangers can also be a source of meaning and happiness. Allow yourself to listen to others with an open mind, reach out to someone who may need it or who feels lonely, or even send them a text message or funny card to check in.

Social Engagement

Your social network can teach you a lot about them, yourself, and the world when you interact with them. There is a lot more to all of us than what is on the surface. Your friends have their own life experiences, acquaintances, travel stories and adventures, strange hobbies, interesting accomplishments, and goals that have not yet been achieved. Let these people into your life and allow yourself to care about them. One of the amazing things about humanity is our ability to care for others, so allow yourself to embrace this quality.

You could even work on your goals with your friends. It would certainly make it easier and more interesting to accomplish them, even providing you with the support to finally complete your goals. Try to be a good listener and friend to the people you care about. In return, a good friend will do the same for you. Share your difficulties with them and face challenges together. Listen to the point of view of other people and see what you can learn about life and relate to. It will also help you see the world in a different way. You are never too old to learn and grow. You may even pick up new, healthy behaviors from your social network. Getting meals with friends and taking part in social dining activities is another great way to promote connectivity and interaction and battle social isolation.

Don't let anyone tell you that you are too old because they are wrong. If you are willing to take the time to put in the work, learn new skills, and approach the world and its people with an open mind, then you will be able to do almost anything you want. Having a social network that is an important part of your life has endless benefits, especially for improving your lifespan and the aging process. They help you enjoy life and can even inspire you to want to carry on living your life to its fullest potential.

MEANINGFUL CONNECTIONS IMPACT LONGEVITY

Having healthy and meaningful relationships with other people doesn't just offer you a variety of mental and physical benefits; they can also have a positive impact on your lifespan. According to Harvard Health Publishing (2011), social relationships have been found to have a positive impact on a person's health by helping them enjoy their daily lives and benefiting their overall well-being. Your relationships with other people are one of the few keys to longevity that encompasses more than a few aspects of your health. Additionally, it doesn't cost you anything to be friendly and connect with other people, so allow yourself to give this strategy a try.

Start by looking at your close friends and family members, even your neighbors. Do your relationships with them make you happier and more content? Or do you perhaps find certain activities that you usually dread—like running errands—more enjoyable simply because your spouse or close friend goes with you? Social relationships will look different depending on the person you are connecting with, as well as whether you are a very social person or not. You may even find that you have a different approach to friendships and people now that you are getting older. It's actually normal because, as you age, your brain changes.

The Brain as You Age

The brain is a social creature, something that can be seen every day. If you aren't a very social person, you may want to deny this, but even people who aren't fans of being around others can still develop meaningful connections. They just look different. Perhaps you have a small group of friends that you are close with, but you also make polite conversation with the cashier when you go grocery shopping. When you are stuck in a queue that feels like it's taking forever, you may find that you start chatting with the people around you, commiserating over the wait time or the heat of the stuffy building. You can even cultivate meaningful relationships with animals like your pet dog, cat, or bird. But the fact remains that our brains are constantly trying to befriend things, be they people or animals.

It's not a bad thing either because social support—even if you are receiving some of that support from a beloved pet—can improve your cardiovascular and mental health, your immune system's functioning, your cognitive health, your life span, and your satisfaction with life (Evans, 2018).

When you experience chronic stress, your body may have high levels of cortisol, which can affect your mental and physical health, especially if it's left untreated. Social relationships have the ability to regulate your stress response system because they provide you with the emotional—and sometimes even physical—support that you need to cope with difficult situations. The brain itself is constantly growing and changing to adapt to and accommodate new situations, thanks to its capacity for neuroplasticity. Neuroplasticity continues as you get older, and it's affected by how you form relationships with other people and form attachments to them. As such, your self-esteem, confidence, physical health, and how your brain adapts form the core of the resilience that you need to survive everyday life and meet the needs of each stage of your life.

As you get older, your short-term memory and quick recall often deteriorate. You may find that it starts to become difficult to remember small things like where you put your car keys or what you had for breakfast the day before. However, this loss is balanced by your increased ability to relate to other people in a compassionate manner. This is believed to result from anxiety's decreased impact on the brain as you get older, allowing you to approach life with more clarity (Evans, 2018).

The brain's ability to adapt and change throughout life allows you to take charge and influence how your mental and physical health and well-being could be impacted. Individuals who have lived over 100 years were found to have had close, meaningful social relationships with others (Evans, 2018). Additionally, getting older helps you become wiser, which results from how you interact with other people and treat them. As a result, cultivating meaningful connections with others can benefit you and your community.

Social Keys to Longevity

Besides earthing, cultivating meaningful connections with other people may be one of the easier anti-aging strategies to access and practice. According to Harvard Health Publishing (2011), the positive impact of social relationships on your lifespan benefits both you and the people you are connecting with. Their impact on your health consists of both biological and behavioral factors. Taking part in caring-behaviors can release stress-reducing hormones and combat the impact of stress on your mind and body. Remember, there are no specific rules or requirements for an activity to qualify as social support. They can range from expressions of affection for your spouse, family member, or friend in the form of a physical hug, kind words, or even a gift that you know will mean something to them, to offering to help them with errands or giving them advice because you already experienced such a situation. There are two main keys to ensuring that your social connections are positively contributing to your lifespan.

Strengthening Your Social Ties

Occasions like holidays, birthdays, or even simply catching up with an old friend are all opportunities to check in with each other. During this time, you can share your ideas, laugh together, or provide them with support and advice. Someone who cares about you will also provide you with the exact same support. You don't have to be friends with everyone. Take the time to focus on the relationships that are meaningful to you while also keeping an open mind. Sometimes, new friends come into our lives in unexpected ways, but they also make them better. Perhaps you could do an activity together, like run errands, or take part in the same hobbies as a book club or volunteering. These activities should make you both happy and allow you to strengthen your relationship for the future.

Remember What Matters to You

The quality of your relationships with other people is more important than the number of friends you have.

You could be a single man or woman and still be able to have meaningful relationships with a close group of friends. Don't let other people tell you that you are too old, need more friends, or have to stop living your life just because you reached a certain age. If you put your mind to it, then you can do it. It's the quality of your life and relationships that matter. Being in a satisfying marriage, or marital-type relationship, can lower your risk of illnesses like cardiovascular disease, while negative interactions with your family or friends could be harmful to your health (Harvard Health Publishing, 2011). Yes, having a social network is important, but your relationships should make you happy and positively impact your life in order to make a difference.

Not everyone is a social butterfly, and you don't have to be. The relationships that you do have with the current people and animals in your life can be just as important and impactful as having a large group of friends and family who care about you. Take the time to reflect on your current relationships with family, friends, spouses, and even old acquaintances. Determine which relationships are beneficial to you and which ones cause you more harm than good. Building meaningful connections with others is just as important as cutting off relationships that hurt you.

HOW TO BUILD MEANINGFUL CONNECTIONS

As you get older, you may find that meeting new people and developing friendships isn't as easy as it was when you were younger. Don't let that stop you. You don't have to give in to the stereotype that getting older is lonely. Meeting new people and developing meaningful friendships is possible if you are willing to put in the effort. First, I want you to ask yourself the following two questions:

- From the people in your life (family, friends, and acquaintances), who gives you the validation, support, and encouragement you need to face challenges and enjoy your life?
- From this group of people, how many of your relationships can be considered quality friendships? You can include spouses and family members here too.

By answering these questions, you give yourself a starting point that will help you determine where to go from here. They may even create more questions that will help you identify what you want to get out of your relationships with other people. Do you first need to work on strengthening the current relationships in your life, or can you start making new friends? Your answers will differ; as such, how you use the strategies that can help you build meaningful connections will also look different.

Strategies That Can Help You Cultivate Meaningful Connections

There are numerous strategies that you can use to cultivate meaningful connections with other people. The list included in this section is not all-inclusive, but it does contain some great suggestions that you can use as a starting point to improve your friendships and build new ones. You may even come up with your own ideas. Write a list of ideas down in your notebook that contains activities that allow you to do something you enjoy, while also helping you bond with friends and family, or even meet new people. Some of these methods have already been mentioned in this guide, but this list—as originally explained by Hartzell (2021)—will give you a bit more detail on how to apply these activities, specifically in terms of cultivating meaningful connections.

Reconnect With Old Friends

Did you have a group of friends that you were close with once, but you just seemed to drift apart from them? Well, now is the perfect time to reach out to them and check-in. You don't have to become best friends. After all, it has been some time, and you have both changed, but give it a chance and see where catching up takes you. You were friends for a reason, you just need to determine if that reason was good enough to pursue a friendship, or even an acquaintance, with them again. Social media sites—like Facebook, Instagram, and Twitter—are great ways to look for your old friends and reconnect. You could start out by sending a simple message that says you have been thinking of them lately and hope that they are doing well. If they respond positively to your message, you can continue chatting with them. You may even reach a point where you are comfortable inviting them out for a cup of coffee or lunch to catch up in person. Go slow, but see where it takes you.

Reach Out to Friends of Friends

Have you ever been sort-of friends with someone because you have a mutual friend? It could be a good idea to reach out to them. You may find that the people you meet through your friends can be interesting people who also share similar interests to you. Already having a mutual friend means that you have something in common with each other. It's now time to reach out directly to this friend-of-a-friend and try to get to know them better. After being introduced, start out simple. Let them know that you have only been told good things about them. You can make polite small talk from here about something your mutual friend may have mentioned. When you go to functions—even if it's lunch with your friend—and you meet them again, make the effort to check in with them and follow up with something they mentioned the last time you saw each other. Going to the same events provides you with a low-pressure environment to interact with a number of people who are familiar, even if you aren't good friends. This counts as a positive social interaction.

Take Part in Online Communities

Technology and social media have made some big advancements in recent years, and they continue to do so. Use this to your advantage. Join an online community where you can meet and interact with a variety of different people. You won't always become best friends, but these interactions can be as meaningful and fulfilling as the relationships you have in real life. Social media is also set up in a way that makes it easy to search for and meet people who have similar interests, hobbies, and professions as you. This can make it easier to interact with strangers because you already have a common interest. Hartzell (2021), found that the following apps are a great additional way to meet new people:

- Meet My Dog
- BumbleBFF
- Friender
- NextDoor

You have to keep in mind that online communities require the same amount of intention and effort on your part that cultivating a physical friendship would. Allow yourself to approach this strategy with an open mind, and be kind and curious as you meet new people.

Join One or Two Local Groups

Joining a local group in your community can be a great way to meet new people who live nearby. Attend at least three or four meetings before deciding whether you want to commit to this group or leave. Local groups could include a religious group, an online community group, volunteering, or even attending classes to learn a new skill. It doesn't matter what you choose. As long as you intentionally interact with the group and try to connect with other members, you will experience some great benefits. The topic of the group gives you a great starting point to initiate small talk with its members. You may need to be the one to initiate conversion, but you might find that you get along great with the other person. If you want to get to know more about them, ask them if they are comfortable exchanging their email address or cell phone number with you. That way, you can arrange to meet outside of the group to get to know each other better.

Get a New Hobby

Combining your "want" to learn something new with cultivating meaningful connections is a great way to attend to more than one need at a time. Ensure that you pursue a hobby that interests you. It may even be something that you have been wanting to do for years. This will also help you fill your spare time and fight off loneliness by bringing a group of people with similar interests together to learn and grow. You could even think about signing up for a class, especially if the hobby is a team sport or requires a bit more technique than can be taught from a book or instructional video. Classes also help you meet people who are passionate about the same topic, regardless of their age. Such hobbies could include cycling, skiing, knitting, scrapbooking, learning an instrument, painting, or even pottery.

Book Club

I've mentioned it before, and it really is a great way to interact with new people. While geared towards literary lovers, a book club can help you meet and connect with a number of different people who all have something interesting to bring to the group. Book clubs are often advertised at bookstores, libraries, and online. Many of the clubs are diverse in the topics or genres they focus on, so find the club that is geared towards your interests. If you can't find a club you are comfortable joining, consider starting your book club. Get family and friends to join you and advertise your club online. You would be surprised at how happy others may be at your initiative to start a book club. You will need to decide where you will meet, the types of books you will read, the best time of day to meet, as well as other factors—like everyone contributes snacks and drinks for each meeting. Don't be afraid to go after the things you have always wanted to pursue.

Volunteer

Again, I have mentioned this activity multiple times throughout this guide. That just shows the type of impact this activity can make on your life. Besides making a difference and giving back to your community, you have the opportunity to meet and interact with new people with the same passions as you, learn new skills, and put your current knowledge and skills to use. When choosing where or how you would like to volunteer, reflect on your skills and experience. What are you passionate about? Would you feel more comfortable volunteering at an animal shelter, or would you prefer something calmer, like volunteering at your local library? The choice is ultimately up to you, but you have to take the time to identify what will make you happy and what you intend to do about it. You could even volunteer at a variety of different events in your community to help you decide what you enjoy. Be sure to give each activity at least a month before you move on to the next one.

It can be daunting to make new friends as you get older, especially if you befriend people who are a bit older or younger than you. However, that doesn't make your friendships any less valuable or meaningful. Friendships can give your life a surprising amount of meaning and purpose. They can make you happy and transform boring, ordinary tasks into an adventure. Each relationship in your life will impact you in a uniquely different way and teach you something about yourself and the world. Allow yourself to open up and give others a chance because you deserve to receive just as much love and happiness as you can give.

KEY TAKEAWAYS

- Meaningful connections have a positive impact on your mental and physical health.
- This important anti-aging technique is often overlooked or even ignored.
- Your sense of self-worth, self-esteem, and confidence is improved through meaningful social relationships.
- It provides you with opportunities to connect and interact with others, as well as allowing for an exchange of support to occur between members in such friendships.
- Social relationships can improve your lifespan.
- The brain changes as you get older, growing with each meaningful connection you make and benefiting both you and your community.
- You need to learn how to cultivate and nurture your relationships with others.
- There are a number of strategies for building meaningful connections with other people. You need to choose what works best for you.

While often overlooked, meaningful connections with other people can provide you with a range of benefits that impact your overall well-being. It's okay if you feel nervous while practicing these strategies, what matters is that you are doing it anyway. Go slow, keep your mind open, and embrace the possibility of new friendships. There is more to anti-aging than ensuring you are mentally and physically healthy. This chapter has provided you with the final step to managing the effects of aging, feeling more energetic, looking younger, and increasing your vitality. It's now time for you to put these steps into practice.

SPREAD THE WORD!

You have all the tools you need to reverse the effects of aging and make yourself feel younger with every passing day… and that puts you in the perfect position to help me spread the word.

Simply by leaving your honest opinion of this book on Amazon, you'll help guide new readers toward the secrets that will change their lives.

LEAVE A REVIEW!

I dream of helping thousands more people reverse the effects of aging and live life to the fullest well into old age. Thank you for helping me to do that.

Scan the QR code for a quick review!

THE KEY TO LIFE

"When I was five my mother always told me happiness was the key to life. When I went to school they asked me what I wanted to be when I grew up. I wrote down "HAPPY". They told me I didn't understand the assignment. I told them they didn't understand life."

— JOHN LENNON

Happiness is a choice. It sounds simplistic, but it is something anyone can do. Choose Happiness. The best method to being happier is to spend time doing things you really enjoy.

Here are some other simple things to do that can add up and have you saying life is good.

1. Cultivate meaningful connections. This can increase feelings of happiness.
2. Get plenty of sleep every night. This is very important for over all health and quality of life.
3. A small amount of exercise can make a difference, by doing exercises that you enjoy doing you will keep at it. The endorphins can make you feel good. Exercise can reduce

anxiety and stress. It also can bring about a more positive mindset.

4. Learn to appreciate the good things you have in your life. Value your accomplishments, even if they seem small. Do not compare yourself to other people. Remember you are your worst critic. Believe in yourself to gain confidence. If you do not have confidence you will not act to move forward in life.
5. Being helpful to people and acts of kindness will make you feel good about yourself.

CONCLUSION

> *There is a fountain of youth: It is your mind, your talents, the creativity you bring to your life and the lives of people you love. When you learn to tap this source, you will truly have defeated age.*
>
> — SOPHIA LOREN

Aging is always framed as something to be avoided; when in reality, it's not as terrifying as it's made out to be. Getting older is inevitable, but you shouldn't let that stop you from living your life. You are only as old as you feel. The information, tools, and strategies discussed in this guide have provided you with the knowledge you need to successfully pursue anti-aging.

Each chapter discussed important information that was both relevant to the aging process, while also detailing how you can combat it. Understanding the science behind aging in Chapter 1 helped you understand how the aging process works and how you can use this knowledge to your advantage. Knowing what happens to your mind and body as you get older gives you the tools needed—as discussed by the six main anti-aging techniques—to slow down the aging process and help your body keep up with how you feel mentally.

This laid the foundation for chapter two's discussion on a positive attitude and its impact on the aging process. You probably began investigating anti-aging methods because you feel a lot younger than your actual age. This chapter helped you learn how to match your mindset and attitude so that you could believe in yourself and your abilities, especially when others try to convince you otherwise.

Through the use of age-defying supplements, discussed in Chapter 3, you learned how to take care of your mind and body's needs in the form of vitamins and minerals. This is especially important if you struggle to get all the nutrition you need from your diet. Supplements don't reverse the aging process, but they can help you to slow it down and make a positive impact on your overall health—which can be quite important as you get older. Supplements also impact your brain in a good way. The brain's ability to learn and grow, regardless of your age, means it's important to look after its health. Chapter four discussed how neuroplasticity is one of your brain's key characteristics that can increase your energy and vitality. Additionally, it has a number of benefits that can be experienced when correctly harnessed.

Unfortunately, stress can negatively impact the aging process. You experience stress every day, throughout your life. If left untreated, chronic stress can start to severely impact your well-being and accelerate the aging process. Using chapter five to better understand how it impacts your mind and body can help you effectively combat it in a way that suits your lifestyle.

More natural anti-aging strategies take the form of earthing. While you may be skeptical at first, chapter six expanded on the science behind this practice. This ancient health practice is easy to access and helps you slow down the aging process in a more natural manner. Chapter seven discussed meaningful connections as an additional anti-aging technique that takes an interesting approach to improving how you age. Impacting both your mental and physical health, it's important to engage with other people and nurture your relationships. They provide you with support and boost your confidence as you get older. Getting older doesn't mean you have to be lonely.

Armed with the knowledge provided in each chapter, you now have the tools needed to improve your health and well-being as you get older, while also decreasing your risk of developing age-related diseases. Having the ability to positively impact your longevity can give you the opportunity to spend more time with the people you care about, as well as the ability to fully enjoy your life now that you have the experience that you didn't have 20-odd years ago. It's never too late to start taking care of yourself and working to become the best version of you. Retired or working, children or no children—each step, strategy, and tool can be adapted to fit into your lifestyle and goals.

I am in my 70s, but I feel a lot younger than that. Using the anti-aging strategies discussed in this guide, I now have the tools to slow down the aging process and enjoy my life, despite what others may say. Society often believes that getting older means you have to stop living your life, but I know that isn't true. Yes, it will take time before you start experiencing any results, but time and patience can help you use the tools effectively, in a way that allows you to feel and look younger, have more energy, and increase your vitality. After completing this guide, you will be able to immediately start implementing the tools and strategies discussed, integrating them into your life in a way that meets your needs and improves your daily habits, allowing you to join the ranks of other SuperAgers.

Aging may be inevitable, but that doesn't mean you have to sit back and stop living your life. You can age gracefully by using the correct anti-aging strategies and tools, as explained throughout this guide. It will be hard at first, but don't give up because it will be worth it. Armed with the tools and knowledge provided in this guide, you too can experience the anti-aging benefits that I have. If you enjoyed this guidebook, please consider leaving a review on Amazon.

REFERENCES

Abud, G. F., De Carvalho, F. G., Batitucci, G., Travieso, S. G., Bueno Junior, C. R., Barbosa Junior, F., Marchini, J. S., and de Freitas, E. C. (2022). Taurine as a possible anti-aging therapy: A controlled clinical trial on taurine antioxidant activity in women ages 55 to 70. *Nutrition*, 101, 111706. https://doi.org/10.1016/j.nut.2022.111706

Ackerman, C. E. (2018, July 25). *What is neuroplasticity? A psychologist explains [+14 Tools]*. Positive Psychology. https://positivepsychology.com/neuroplasticity/

Admin. (2020). *The 12 best anti-aging supplements*. Lift and Tuck. https://liftandtuck.co.za/2020/04/10/the-12-best-anti-aging-supplements/

Amaresan, S. (2021, April 29). 10 Creative ways to keep a positive attitude no matter *Hub Spot*. https://blog.hubspot.com/service/posi tive-attitude

Anti-aging-Healthy aging. (2012). Earthing Nederland. https://www.earthingnederland.nl/antiaging?Lng=en

Are B12 injections the missing link for anti-aging fight? (2020, January 21). Invigor Medical. https://www.invigormedical.com/anti-aging/are-b12-injections-the-missing-link-for-your-anti-aging-fight/what.

Ayunin, Q., Miatmoko, A., Soeratri, W., Erawati, T., Susanto, J., and Legowo, D. (2022). Improving the anti-ageing activity of coenzyme Q10 through protransfersome-loaded emulgel. *Scientific Reports*, 12(1). https://doi.org/10.1038/s41598-021-04708-4

Bailey, R. (2020). *What does the brain's cerebral cortex do?* ThoughtCo. https://www.thoughtco.com/anatomy-of-the-brain-cerebral-cortex-373217

BD Editors. (2016). Chromosome: Definition, function and structure. In the *Biology Dictionary*. https://biologydictionary.net/chromosome/

Benameur, T., Soleti, R., Panaro, M. A., La Torre, M. E., Monda, V.,

Messina, G., and Porro, C. (2021). Curcumin as prospective anti-aging natural compound: Focus on brain. *National Library of Medicine,* 26(16), 4794. https://doi.org/10.3390/molecules26164794

Berridge, M. J. (2017). Vitamin D deficiency accelerates aging and age-related diseases: a novel hypothesis. *The Journal of Physiology,* 595(22), 6825–6836. https://doi.org/10.1113/jp274887

Betteridge, D. J. (2000). What is oxidative stress? *Metabolism,* 49(2), 3–8. https://doi.org/10.1016/s0026-0495(00)80077-3

Biochemical reactions. (2012, November 15). CK-12 Foundation. https://www.ck12.org/c/physical-science/biochemical-reactions/lesson/Biochemical-Reaction-Chemistry-MS-PS/#

Britannica. (2022). *Homeostasis: Definition, function, examples, and facts.* In Encyclopædia Britannica. https://www.britannica.com/science/homeostasis

BYJU'S Admin. (2020, June 15). *Cortisol hormone - functions, synthesis and hormonal level.* BYJU'S. https://byjus.com/biology/cortisol-hormone/

Cabrera, Á. J. R. (2015). Zinc, aging, and immunosenescence: an overview. *Pathobiology of Aging and Age-Related Diseases,* 5(1), 25592. https://doi.org/10.3402/pba.v5.25592

Cahn, L. (2018, September 19). *Bad stress versus good stress: How to know the difference.* The Healthy. https://www.thehealthy.com/mental-health/stress/bad-stress-vs-good-stress-how-to-know-the-difference/

Cherry, K. (2022). *What is neuroplasticity?* Very Well Mind. https://www.verywellmind.com/what-is-brain-plasticity-2794886

Chevalier, G., Sinatra, S. T., Oschman, J. L., Sokal, K., and Sokal, P. (2012). Earthing: Health implications of reconnecting the human body to the Earth's surface electrons. *Journal of Environmental and Public Health,* 2012, 1–8. https://doi.org/10.1155/2012/291541

Developing a positive attitude. (2017, January 13). *Clarke University.* https://www.clarke.edu/campus-life/health-wellness/counseling/articles-advice/developing-a-positive-attitude/

Codiva, M. (2022, October 8). *Amino acid taurine can be used in anti-aging treatments, study reveals.* Science Times. https://www.science

times.com/articles/40374/20221007/eg-amino-acid-taurine-used-anti-aging-treatments.htm

Cynthiam. (2021, February 26). *A 9-step guide to increase your neuroplasticity (and rewire your brain).* Second Wind Movement. https://secondwindmovement.com/neuroplasticity/

Daniells, S. (2016, November 23). Ashwagandha root extracts shows anti-aging effect: Cell study. *Nutra Ingredients*. https://www.nutraingredients.com/Article/2016/11/23/Ashwagandha-root-extracts-shows-anti-aging-effect-Cell-study

Drinking too much alcohol can harm your health. (2022). Centers for Disease Control and Prevention. https://www.cdc.gov/alcohol/fact-sheets/alcohol-use.htm

DSM. (n.d.). *New ways in anti-aging with folic acid cosmetic benefits and formulation guidelines.* Retrieved October 20, 2022, from https://www.dsm.com/content/dam/protected/personal-care/en_US/vitamins/vitamins_distributor/Folic%20Acid%20for%20Beauty%20Care_Master%20Presentation_2017-04.pdf

Earthing mat. (2014). Grounded.com. https://grounded.com/earthing-mat

Evans, K. (2018, September 17). *Why relationships are the key to longevity.* Mindful. https://www.mindful.org/why-relationships-are-the-key-to-longevity/

5 Ways older adults can reduce stress. (2016, April 4). Judson Senior Living. https://www.judsonsmartliving.org/blog/5-ways-older-adults-can-reduce-stress/

4 Habits of "super agers." (2018, August 28). Northwestern Medicine. https://www.nm.org/healthbeat/healthy-tips/4-habits-super-agers

Frank, M. O., and Caceres, B. A. (2015). Inflammaging: A concept analysis. *The Journal for Nurse Practitioners*, 11(2), 258–261. https://doi.org/10.1016/j.nurpra.2014.08.005

Goldsmith, T. C. (2016). Evolution of aging theories: Why modern programmed aging concepts are transforming medical research. *Biochemistry (Moscow)*, 81(12), 1406–1412. https://doi.org/10.1134/s0006297916120026

Grounding Mat. (2022a). Amazon. https://www.amazon.com/Earthing-Grounding-Reconnect-Recovery-35-4x23-6/dp/

Grounding sleep mat kit. (2022b). Amazon. https://www.amazon.com/Grounding-grounding-earthing-EARTHING-Products/dp/

Hartzell, K. (2021, August 5). *7 Tips for making friends in middle age.* Hartzell Counseling. https://hartzellcounseling.com/7-tips-for-making-friends-in-middle-age/

Harvard T.H. Chan School of Public Health. (2022, August 24). *Positive attitude about aging could boost health.* Harvard. https://www.hsph.harvard.edu/news/hsph-in-the-news/positive-attitude-about-aging-could-boost-health/

Holford, P. (2022, June 13). *The importance of earthing.* Patrick Holford. https://www.patrickholford.com/advice/the-importance-of-earthing/

Home: Quotes. (2020, September 29). Daily Inspirational Quotes. https://www.dailyinspirationalquotes.in/2020/09/dont-worry-about-getting-old-worry-about-thinking-old-unknown/

How your brain thrives on positivity. (2020). *Achieve Medical Center.* https://www.achievemedicalcenter.com/blog-post/your-brain-thrives-on-positivity

Hurst, K. (2017, December 19). *15 Easy positive thinking exercises to do.* The Law of Attraction. https://thelawofattraction.com/positive-thinking-exercises/

Ibe, O. (2022). *What is earthing?* Very Well Mind. https://www.verywellmind.com/what-is-earthing-5220089

Jagoo, K. (2022). *Stress is aging you faster—but it's possible to slow down the biological clock.* Very Well Mind. https://www.verywellmind.com/stress-is-aging-you-faster-but-it-s-possible-to-slow-down-the-biological-clock-5212916

Jeffries, M. (2021, March 20). *Melatonin for skin: The new anti-aging secret? Dr. Michelle Jeffries.* https://drmichellejeffries.com/melatonin-skin/

Keanu Reeves, a different kind of celebrity. (2019, October 14). Exploring Your Mind. https://exploringyourmind.com/keanu-reeves-a-different-kind-of-celebrity/

Kelly, K. (2017, February 21). *The anti-aging benefits of omega-3's*. Rejuvime Medical. https://www.rejuvimemedical.com/blog/the-anti-aging-benefits-of-omega-3s/

Killilea, D. W., and Maier, J. A. M. (2008). A connection between magnesium deficiency and aging: new insights from cellular studies. *Magnesium Research*, 21(2), 77–82. https://www.ncbi.nlm.nih.gov/pmc/articles/PMC2790427/

Kim, M. (2019, November 21). *Secrets of Hollywood's "super-agers" stars*. Orange Twist. https://orangetwist.com/hollywood-superagers/

Layton, J., and Mancini, M. (2008, September 22). *How does the body make electricity—and how does it use it?* HowStuffWorks. https://health.howstuffworks.com/human-body/systems/nervous-system/human-body-make-electricity.htm

Lithium might work as an anti-aging drug, depending on your genes. (2017). King's College London. https://www.kcl.ac.uk/archive/news/ioppn/records/2018/december/lithium-might-work-as-an-anti-aging-drug-depending-on-your-genes

Lockett, E. (2019, August 30). *Grounding: Exploring earthing science and the benefits behind it*. Healthline. https://www.healthline.com/health/grounding#the-science

Loren, S. (2015). *Sophia Loren quotes (author of Yesterday, Today, Tomorrow)*. Goodreads. https://www.goodreads.com/author/quotes/290913.Sophia_Loren

Ma, L., Liu, Q., Tian, M., Tian, X., and Gao, L. (2021). Mechanisms of melatonin in anti-aging and its regulation effects in radiation-induced premature senescence. *Radiation Medicine and Protection*, 2(1), 33–37. https://doi.org/10.1016/j.radmp.2021.01.003

Macmillan, L. (2022, May 16). *The science of longevity*. Vanderbilt Medicine; Vanderbilt University. https://medschool.vanderbilt.edu/vanderbilt-medicine/the-science-of-longevity/

Mayer Robinson, K. (2021, March 24). *Supplements and aging*. Compass by WebMD; WebMD. https://www.webmd.com/healthy-aging/features/supplements-aging

McCray, D. (2022a). *Quote: Never lose the sense of optimism you had as a youth, it'll help keep you young*. (Original work published 2022)

McCray, D. (2022b). *Quote: You do better in life if you have an open mind because it lets you think outside of the box.* (Original work published 2022)

Merriam-Webster. (n.d.-a). Biological clock. In the *Merriam-Webster Dictionary*. Retrieved October 26, 2022, from https://www.merriam-webster.com/dictionary/biological%20clock

Merriam-Webster. (n.d.-b). Craniosacral therapy. In the *Merriam-Webster Dictionary*. Retrieved October 27, 2022, from https://www.merriam-webster.com/dictionary/craniosacral%20therapy

Merriam-Webster. (n.d.-c). Endocrine system. In the *Merriam-Webster Dictionary*. Retrieved October 14, 2022, from https://www.merriam-webster.com/medical/endocrine%20system

Merriam-Webster. (n.d.-d). Free radicals. In the *Merriam-Webster Dictionary*. Retrieved October 14, 2022, from https://www.merriam-webster.com/dictionary/free%20radicals

Merriam-Webster. (n.d.-e). Gene. In the *Merriam-Webster Dictionary*. Retrieved October 14, 2022, from https://www.merriam-webster.com/dictionary/gene

Merriam-Webster. (n.d.-f). Innate immunity. In the *Merriam-Webster Dictionary*. Retrieved October 26, 2022, from https://www.merriam-webster.com/medical/innate%20immunity

Merriam-Webster. (n.d.-g). Ion. In the *Merriam-Webster Dictionary*. Retrieved October 28, 2022, from https://www.merriam-webster.com/dictionary/ion

Merriam-Webster. (n.d.-h). Macrophage. In the *Merriam-Webster Dictionary*. Retrieved October 26, 2022, from https://www.merriam-webster.com/dictionary/macrophage

Merriam-Webster. (n.d.-i). Massage. In the *Merriam-Webster Dictionary*. Retrieved October 27, 2022, from https://www.merriam-webster.com/dictionary/massage

Merriam-Webster. (n.d.-j). Metabolism. In the *Merriam-Webster Dictionary*. Retrieved October 14, 2022, from https://www.merriam-webster.com/dictionary/metabolism

Merriam-Webster. (n.d.-k). Mitochondria. In the *Merriam-Webster Dictionary*. Retrieved October 14, 2022, from https://www.

merriam-webster.com/dictionary/mitochondria

Merriam-Webster. (n.d.-l). Reiki. In the *Merriam-Webster Dictionary*. Retrieved October 27, 2022, from https://www.merriam-webster.com/dictionary/Reiki

Merriam-Webster. (n.d.-m). Tai Chi. In the *Merriam-Webster Dictionary*. Retrieved October 27, 2022, from https://www.merriam-webster.com/dictionary/tai%20chi

Merriam-Webster. (n.d.-n). Yoga. In the *Merriam-Webster Dictionary*. Retrieved October 27, 2022, from https://www.merriam-webster.com/dictionary/yoga

Modified citrus pectin (MCP). (2022). Cancer Research UK. https://www.cancerresearchuk.org/about-cancer/cancer-in-general/treatment/complementary-alternative-therapies/individual-therapies/modified-citrus-pectin-mcp

Neuroplasticity. (2019). Psychology Today. https://www.psychologytoday.com/us/basics/neuroplasticity

Nunez, K. (2021, March 23). *Why do we get old?* Healthline. https://www.healthline.com/health/why-do-we-age

Ohio State University. (2012). *Omega-3 supplements may slow a biological effect of aging*. Science Daily. https://www.sciencedaily.com/releases/2012/10/121001140957.htm

Raguraman, V., and Subramaniam, J. R. (2016). Withania somnifera root extract enhances telomerase activity in the human HeLa cell line. *Advances in Bioscience and Biotechnology*, 07(04), 199–204. https://doi.org/10.4236/abb.2016.74018

Roberts, R. (2022, May 13). *A "longevity success story": Canada's growing 85-plus group makes us wonder what the key is to healthy aging*. Healthing.ca. https://www.healthing.ca/wellness/aging/a-longevity-success-story-canadas-growing-85-plus-group-makes-us-wonder-whats-the-key-to-healthy-aging

Roser, M., Ortiz-Ospina, E., and Ritchie, H. (2019, October). *Life expectancy*. Our World in Data. https://ourworldindata.org/life-expectancy

Ruscio, M. (2021, October 29). *Modified citrus pectin: Your guide to benefits, risks, and usage*. Dr. Ruscio. https://drruscio.com/modified-citrus-pectin/

Salters-Pedneault, K. (2022). *What is serotonin and how does it regulate bodily functions?* Very Well Mind. https://www.verywellmind.com/what-is-serotonin-425327

Salvador, L., Singaravelu, G., Harley, C. B., Flom, P., Suram, A., and Raffaele, J. M. (2016). A natural product telomerase activator lengthens telomeres in humans: A randomized, double blind, and placebo controlled study. *Rejuvenation Research*, 19(6), 478–484. https://doi.org/10.1089/rej.2015.1793

Sengupta, A. (2021, August 12). *Top 10 Hollywood celebrities that don't seem to age*. Sportskeeda. https://www.sportskeeda.com/pop-culture/top-10-hollywood-celebrities-age

Sharing knowledge quotes (8 quotes). (n.d.). Goodreads | Meet your next favorite book. https://www.goodreads.com/quotes/tag/sharing-knowledge

Simes, D. C., Viegas, C. S. B., Araújo, N., and Marreiros, C. (2019). Vitamin K as a powerful micronutrient in aging and age-related diseases: Pros and cons from clinical studies. *International Journal of Molecular Sciences*, 20(17), 4150. https://doi.org/10.3390/ijms20174150

Smith, G. S. (2013). Aging and neuroplasticity. *Dialogues in Clinical Neuroscience*, 15(1), 3–5. https://doi.org/10.31887/dcns.2013.15.1/gsmith

Sohn, E.-J., Kim, J. M., Kang, S.-H., Kwon, J., An, H. J., Sung, J.-S., Cho, K. A., Jang, I.-S., and Choi, J.-S. (2018). Restoring effects of natural antioxidant quercetin on cellular senescent human dermal fibroblasts. *The American Journal of Chinese Medicine*, 46(04), 853–873. https://doi.org/10.1142/s0192415x18500453

Splichal, E. (n.d.). *Anti-aging effects of earthing*. NABOSO. https://irp-cdn.multiscreensite.com/9bf295cf/files/uploaded/Anti-Aging%20Effects%20of%20Earthing.pdf

Stancu, A. L. (2015). AMPK activation can delay aging. *Discoveries*, 3(4), e53. https://doi.org/10.15190/d.2015.45

Strengthen relationships for longer, healthier life. (2011, January 18). Harvard Health Publishing. https://www.health.harvard.edu/health

beat/strengthen-relationships-for-longer-healthier-life

Stress management: Important at any age. (2021, August 8). Johns Hopkins Medicine. https://www.hopkinsmedicine.org/health/wellness-and-prevention/stress-management-important-at-any-age

The Benefits and effects of carditone. (2019). MedFriendly Medical Blog. https://blog.medfriendly.com/2019/05/the-benefits-and-effects-of-carditone.html

The importance of meaningful relationships. (2020, May 15). The Carrington at Lincolnwood. https://www.thecarrington.com/2020/05/15/importance-of-meaningful-relationships/

The importance of neuroplasticity as we age. (2021, June). Better Aging. https://www.betteraging.com/aging-science/the-importance-of-neuroplasticity-as-we-age/

The importance of a positive mental attitude. (2019, March 26). Pure Recovery California. https://purerecoveryca.com/the-importance-of-a-positive-mental-attitude/

Thiele, T. (2022). *Understanding electrical grounding and how it works.* The Spruce. https://www.thespruce.com/what-is-grounding-1152859

van Deursen, J. M. (2019). Senolytic therapies for healthy longevity. *Science,* 364(6441), 636–637. https://doi.org/10.1126/science.aaw1299

WebMD Editorial Contributors. (2020). *The benefits of vitamin C for your skin.* Radiance by WebMD. https://www.webmd.com/beauty/ss/slideshow-benefits-of-vitamin-c-for-skin

WebMD Editorial Contributors, and Vogin, G. D. (2002, February 26). *Myth vs. reality on anti-aging vitamins.* Radiance by WebMD. https://www.webmd.com/beauty/features/myth-vs-reality-on-anti-aging-vitamins

Weschawalit, S., Thongthip, S., Phutrakool, P., and Asawanonda, P. (2017). Glutathione and its antiaging and antimelanogenic effects. *Clinical, Cosmetic and Investigational Dermatology,* Volume 10, 147–153. https://doi.org/10.2147/ccid.s128339

What's a super-ager? (2017, October 11). El Camino Health. https://www.elcaminohealth.org/stay-healthy/blog/whats-super-ager

Whelan, C., and Santos-Longhurst, A. (2022, March 25). The Benefits

— and limits — of vitamin A for your skin. Healthline. https://www.healthline.com/health/beauty-skincare/vitamin-a-for-skin

Wilson, J. (2014, April 30). *Brain anti-aging: 9 Steps to better neuroplasticity*. Remedy Grove. https://remedygrove.com/wellness/Brain-Training-Improve-Your-Neuroplasticity-with-10-Easy-Tips

Woolston, C. (2021). Aging and stress. In *Health Day*. Consumer Health News. https://consumer.healthday.com/encyclopedia/aging-1/age-health-news-7/aging-and-stress-645997.html

Wu, L. E., and Sinclair, D. A. (2016). Restoring stem cells — all you need is NAD+. *Cell Research*, 26(9), 971–972. https://doi.org/10.1038/cr.2016.80

Yegorov, Y. E., Poznyak, A. V., Nikiforov, N. G., Sobenin, I. A., and Orekhov, A. N. (2020). The Link between Chronic Stress and Accelerated Aging. *Biomedicines*, 8(7), 198. https://doi.org/10.3390/biomedicines8070198

Yelland, E., Hosier, A. F., and Traywick, L. S. (2015). *Keys to embracing aging: Positive attitude*. Frontier District Kansas State University. https://www.frontierdistrict.k-state.edu/family/keys-to-embracing-aging/fact_sheets/Positive%20Attitude.pdf

What is Earthing? (2017). Yogapedia. https://www.yogapedia.com/definition/10627/earthing#

www.ingramcontent.com/pod-product-compliance
Ingram Content Group UK Ltd.
Pitfield, Milton Keynes, MK11 3LW, UK
UKHW062308290726
14090UKWH00018B/952

9 798988 369202